LOW CARB RECIPES COOKBOOK

2100 Days of Delicious Recipes with Pictures to Guide You Through a Journey of Health and Taste

By

Michael C. Gillum

Copyright© By Michael C. Gillum, 2024

All rights reserved. Unauthorized duplication or distribution of this material in any form is strictly prohibited. No part of this publication may be reproduced, stored in a retrieval system, or transmitted in any form or by any means, electronic, mechanical, photocopying, recording, or otherwise, without prior written permission from the publisher.

Table of content

INTRODUCTION **6**

CHAPTER 1 : THE CONCEPT BEHIND THE LOW-CARB AND HIGH-PROTEIN DIET **8**

CHAPTER 2: BENEFITS OF A HIGH PROTEIN, LOW CARB DIET **12**

CHAPTER 3 : BREAKFAST RECIPES **14**

Egg-cellent Veggie Scramble 14
Avocado Delight Breakfast Bowl 15
Bacon & Spinach Omelette Roll 16
Keto Cauliflower Hash Browns 17
Smoked Salmon & Cream Cheese Wraps 18
Zucchini Fritters with Sour Cream Dip 19
Almond Flour Pancakes with Berries 20
Mediterranean Egg Muffins 21
Chia Seed Pudding Parfait 22
Greek Yogurt Breakfast Smoothie 23
Keto Coconut Porridge 24
Turkey Sausage Breakfast Skillet 25
Cucumber and Cream Cheese Sandwiches 26
Cauliflower Crust Quiche Bites 27
Almond Butter Banana Smoothie 28
Spinach and Mushroom Breakfast Casserole 28
Coconut Flour Waffles with Whipped Cream 29
Low-Carb Breakfast Burrito Bowl 30
Broccoli and Cheese Egg Muffins 30
Peanut Butter Protein Balls 31

CHAPTER 4 : BREAD RECIPES **32**

Flaxseed Almond Bread 32
Coconut Flour Zucchini Bread 33
Keto Cloud Bread Rolls 34
Chia Seed Psyllium Husk Bread 35
Low-Carb Cauliflower Breadsticks 35
Sesame Seed Keto Bread Loaf 36
Cheese and Herb Keto Biscuits 37
Almond Flour Rosemary Focaccia 38
Pumpkin Seed Flax Bread 38
Spinach and Feta Cheese Bread 39
Sunflower Seed Keto Flatbread 40
Walnut Flour Banana Bread 41

CHAPTER 5 : APPETIZERS RECIPES **42**

Cucumber and Cream Cheese Bites 42
Bacon-Wrapped Asparagus Spears 42
Keto Caprese Skewers 43
Avocado Stuffed with Tuna Salad 43
Zucchini Parmesan Chips 44

Buffalo Cauliflower Bites 45

Mini Bell Pepper Nachos 45

Spinach and Artichoke Dip Stuffed Mushrooms 46

Smoked Salmon Cucumber Rolls 47

Deviled Eggs with Avocado 47

Greek Yogurt Ranch Veggie Dip Cups 48

Spicy Chicken Lettuce Wraps 48

CHAPTER 6 : SALAD & SOUPS RECIPES **50**

Grilled Chicken Caesar Salad 50

Avocado and Bacon Spinach Salad 51

Greek Salad with Feta and Olives 52

Shrimp and Avocado Cobb Salad 52

Broccoli Cauliflower Salad with Lemon Dressing 53

Thai Beef Salad with Peanut Dressing 54

Caprese Salad with Balsamic Glaze 55

Taco Salad with Ground Turkey 55

Creamy Cauliflower Soup with Crispy Bacon 56

Chicken Zoodle Soup 57

Tomato Basil Soup with Parmesan Crisps 57

Spinach and Sausage Soup 58

Keto Broccoli Cheese Soup 59

Spicy Thai Coconut Chicken Soup 59

Mexican Chicken Avocado Lime Soup 60

Creamy Mushroom Soup with Garlic and Thyme 61

CHAPTER 7 : SIDE DISHES RECIPES **62**

Garlic Butter Roasted Brussels Sprouts 62

Parmesan Roasted Asparagus Spears 62

Cauliflower Mash with Chives 63

Lemon Garlic Green Beans 64

Cheesy Baked Zucchini Sticks 64

Creamy Spinach and Mushroom Gratin 65

Roasted Garlic Cauliflower Rice 66

Broccoli Bacon Salad with Creamy Dressing 66

Lemon Herb Grilled Eggplant 67

Balsamic Glazed Brussels Sprouts 68

Cheesy Baked Cauliflower Tots 68

Sauteed Garlic Butter Mushrooms 69

Green Bean Almondine 70

Rosemary Roasted Radishes 70

Creamy Dijon Brussels Sprouts 71

Lemon Parmesan Roasted Broccoli 72

Spaghetti Squash Au Gratin 72

Mediterranean Cucumber Salad 73

BACON-WRAPPED GREEN BEAN BUNDLES 74

Creamy Garlic Parmesan Spaghetti Squash 75

CHAPTER 8 : MAIN DISHES RECIPES **76**

Lemon Garlic Butter Salmon 76

Keto Beef and Broccoli Stir-Fry 76

Cauliflower Crust Pizza with Pepperoni 77

Grilled Chicken with Avocado Salsa 78

Zucchini Noodles with Pesto and Cherry Tomatoes 79

Low-Carb Eggplant Lasagna 79

Turkey and Spinach Stuffed Portobello Mushrooms 80

Shrimp Scampi with Zoodles 81

Keto Butter Chicken 82

Stuffed Bell Peppers with Ground Turkey and Quinoa 83

Spaghetti Squash Carbonara 84

Baked Lemon Herb Chicken Thighs 85

Cauliflower Fried Rice with Shrimp 85

Greek Turkey Meatballs with Tzatziki Sauce 86

Coconut Curry Salmon with Cauliflower Rice 87

Beef and Cauliflower Skillet Hash 88

Creamy Garlic Parmesan Chicken Thighs 89

Mexican Cauliflower Rice Bowl 89

Teriyaki Tofu Stir-Fry with Broccoli 90

Pork Tenderloin with Dijon Mustard Sauce 91

Chicken Alfredo with Zucchini Noodles 92

Sesame Ginger Beef Stir-Fry 92

Creamy Tuscan Chicken with Spinach and Sun-Dried Tomatoes 93

Spicy Cajun Shrimp with Cauliflower Grits 94

Baked Cod with Lemon Herb Butter 95

Low-Carb Chicken Fajita Bowl 95

Beef and Mushroom Skewers with Chimichurri Sauce 96

Turkey and Cauliflower Shepherd's Pie 97

Lemon Garlic Butter Shrimp Scampi 98

Thai Basil Chicken Stir-Fry 98

Keto BBQ Ribs with Coleslaw 99

Eggplant Parmesan with Marinara Sauce 100

Grilled Lemon Herb Chicken Breasts 101

Moroccan Spiced Lamb Chops with Cauliflower Couscous 101

Coconut Lime Shrimp with Cauliflower Rice 102

Beef and Cabbage Stir-Fry 103

Stuffed Chicken Breast with Spinach and Feta 104

Baked Pesto Chicken with Cherry Tomatoes 105

Spicy Tofu and Vegetable Stir-Fry 106

Lemon Herb Grilled Pork Chops 107

CHAPTER 9 : DESSERTS RECIPES **108**

Keto Chocolate Avocado Mousse 108

Low-Carb Strawberry Cheesecake Bites 108

Almond Flour Lemon Poppy Seed Cake 109

Coconut Flour Chocolate Chip Cookies 110

Sugar-Free Blueberry Chia Seed Pudding 110

Chocolate Peanut Butter Fat Bombs 111

Vanilla Bean Greek Yogurt Panna Cotta 112

Raspberry Almond Flour Cake Bars 112

No-Bake Peanut Butter Chocolate Bars 113

Keto Coconut Macaroons 114
Avocado Chocolate Fudge Brownies.. 114
Lemon Ricotta Cheesecake Muffins 116

CONCLUSION.. 117

INTRODUCTION

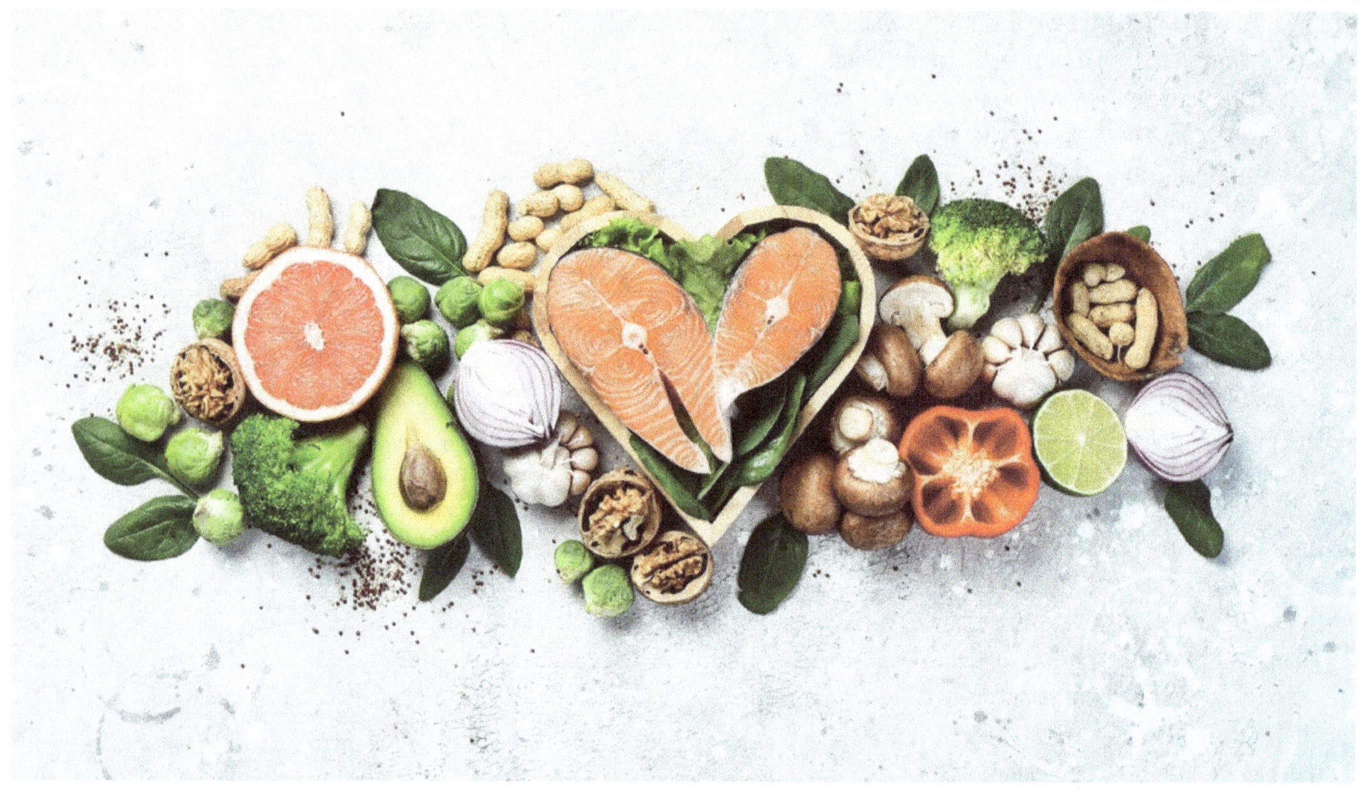

In the realm of low-carb cookery, tasty tastes and healthful eating coexist! We cordially encourage you to peruse this book's wealth of delectable recipes, which prioritize careful nutrition and healthy ingredients without compromising flavor or delight.

Because of their possible health advantages—weight reduction, better blood sugar management, and higher energy levels—low-carb diets have become increasingly popular in recent years. Reducing carbohydrate consumption and emphasizing whole foods high in nutrients provide a novel viewpoint on sustainable and pleasurable healthy eating.

Regardless of your level of expertise with low-carb cooking, this cookbook is meant to motivate and encourage you at every stage of your quest. Every meal, from filling breakfasts to filling lunches, from tasty dinners to decadent desserts, is painstakingly developed to provide taste, texture, and nutritional content.

But this book is a celebration of the rich tastes and creative opportunities that are abundant in low-carb cooking, not just a compilation of recipes. The wide range of foods offered here, covering many countries, cuisines, and dietary requirements, offers something for everyone to like.

There are plenty of choices to please your palate and nourish your body, whether you're in the mood for a rich piece of chocolate avocado mousse cake, a spicy Mediterranean salad, or a cosy bowl of cauliflower mac and cheese.

We are here to empower you with information, advice, and tools to help you succeed on your low-carb journey. However, go beyond the recipes. We'll provide you with the information and direction you need to make educated decisions and meet your health and wellness objectives, from meal planning techniques to ingredient swaps.

So as you set out on this gastronomic voyage, we want you to relish the moment, welcome your inventiveness, and relish the path to a happier, healthier self. These recipes should provide you pleasure and inspiration in the kitchen whether you're cooking for yourself, your family, or your friends.

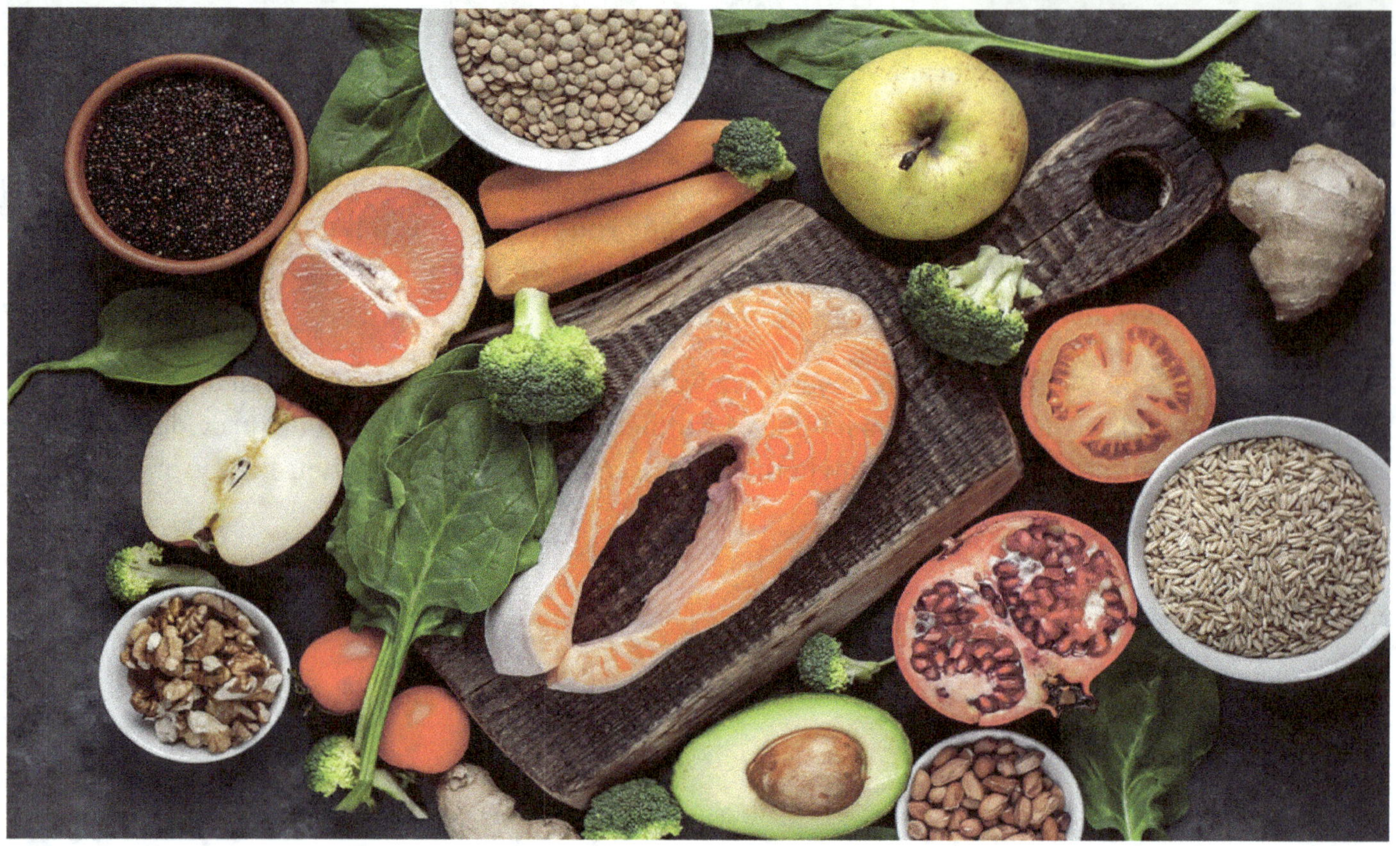

Low-carb, high-protein diets restrict carbs and emphasize protein. Like other diets, including the ketogenic diet, a high-protein, low-carb diet has no universal meaning. People who adhere to it may thus consume different ratios of macronutrients.

A "low-carb" diet includes less than 130 grammes of carbohydrates daily or less than 26% of total calories from carbohydrates. 130 grammes is not much more than 8.5 bread slices. Higher protein diets provide more protein than the recommended daily allowance (RDA), now 0.8 grammes per kilogramme of body weight or 0.36 grammes per pound. This equates to 10% of daily calories for a 2,000-calorie diet or 54 grams of protein for a 150-pound person. Most high-protein diets include between 1.8 and 3 grammes of protein per kilogramme of body weight per day or between 0.8 and 1.36 grammes per pound of body weight daily.

Applying this to your present menu: Forty per cent of the calories in a 2,000-calorie diet may come from protein, twenty-five per cent from carbs, and thirty-five per cent from fat. This works out to be around 1.4 grams of protein per pound, or 200 grams of protein and 125 grams of carbs for a 150-pound person.

However, the high-protein, low-carb dietary pattern is flexible, so some people may eat more protein and fewer carbs and others less protein and more carbohydrates.

The Importance of Protein.

Prior to exploring the potential benefits of eating low-carb, high-protein, it's important to remember that some experts argue that "high" protein diets should really be regarded as standard protein diets.

This is because most people need the very minimal amount of protein—the RDA—to maintain basic health needs include preventing muscle loss and obtaining enough nitrogen.

This suggests that certain "high" protein diets might really be more near to optimum for most people, especially those who need more protein, including pregnant women, physically active people, and older persons.

Reducing or limiting carbohydrate intake frees up more room for meals heavy in protein and usually means eating fewer of the highly processed, refined-carbohydrate snack items and sweets.

List Of High-Protein, Low-Carb Foods

ANIMAL PROTEIN

Animal meals usually provide the most grams of protein per serving than other protein sources, and animal proteins are carb-free. If all you are looking for is high-protein meals, these are the best.

CHICKEN

The sort of meat and cooking technique used in a chicken dinner may significantly affect the macronutrient makeup of the meal. But according to FoodData Central, 100 grammes (about 3.5 ounces) of skinless, boneless chicken breast cooked without seasonings has 32.1 grams of protein and 0 grams of carbohydrates.

BEEF

How beef is diced and cooked affects its macronutrient profiles, just as with chicken. FoodData Central reports that a 100-gramme piece of 90% lean ground beef has 0 grammes of carbohydrates and 18.2 grammes of protein.

PORK

According to FoodData Central, a 100-gram lean pork tenderloin roasted without any additional spices provides 0 grams of carbohydrates and 26.2 grams of protein.

DUCK

A 100-gramme portion of roasted duck meat from a home farm has 0 grammes of carbs and 23.5 grammes of protein.

JERKY

Jerky snacks are excellent when you need a high-protein, non-refrigerated snack to get you through until your next meal. 100 grams of beef jerky with dry flavor (salt and pepper, for instance) contains 33.2 grams of protein.

DAIRY

Dairy products give much protein to those who can tolerate lactose. Plenty of calcium is also found in dairy products!

MILK

One gramme of protein equals one ounce, or eight grammes, in a cup of whole milk. A serving of one cup each of nonfat and low-fat (2%) milk has 8.5 grammes of protein. But whether milk is "low-carb" for you depends on how much carbs you can tolerate: Depending on the variety, an 8-ounce glass of milk contains 12 to 13 grammes of carbohydrates.

GREEK YOGURT

For every 100 grams, plain nonfat Greek yogurt has more than 10 grams of protein and less than 4 grams of carbohydrates. In comparison, the protein content of full-fat plain Greek yogurt is slightly less than 9 grams per 100 grams, while the carbohydrates are almost 5 grams.

COTTAGE CHEESE

For every 100 grams, low-fat cottage cheese has 11 grams of protein and just 4 grams of carbohydrates. In comparison, full-fat cottage cheese has 4.6 grams of carbohydrates and 11.6 grams of protein.

MOZZARELLA CHEESE

FoodData Central reports that 100 grams of mozzarella cheese contains an astounding 23.7 grams of protein and just 4.4 grams of carbohydrates. Because of this, mozzarella cheese is among the dairy products with the most significant protein content.

FISH AND SEAFOOD

Some fish and shellfish provide you with a lot of protein and none in terms of carbs.

SALMON

Per 100 grammes, smoked Chinook salmon has 18.3 grammes of protein and 0 grammes of carbs.

TUNA

Fresh, cooked bluefin tuna has zero carbohydrates and 29.9 grams of protein per 100 grammes. But to enjoy these advantages, fresh tuna is not necessary! There are 19 grammes of protein in every 100 grammes of canned light tuna.

TILAPIA

For every 100 grams of cooked tilapia, there are almost 26 grams of protein and zero grams of carbohydrates.

TROUT

According to FoodData Central, rainbow trout raised on farms have slightly less protein per 100 grams (19.9 grammes) than rainbow trout collected in the wild, which has 20.5 grammes.

PLANT FOODS

There are few plant-based protein sources that can match animal protein sources in terms of protein and carbohydrate composition. For example, although whole grains are often mentioned as a healthy source of protein, they are by no means low in carbohydrates.

PEANUT BUTTER

Although a 100-gram portion of peanut butter has 14% of its calories from carbs, it is a high-protein plant meal. That amounts to 22 grammes of carbohydrates. Furthermore, protein accounts for 14% of calories, higher than many plant-based diets.

TOFU

Like animal proteins, the way tofu is prepared—firm, medium, soft, or light tofu—dramatically alters its nutritional profile. The brand may also impact it. The USDA states that for every 100 grammes of firm tofu, there are 17.3 grammes of protein and 2.78 grammes of carbohydrates.

TEMPEH

Similar to tofu, tempeh is a fermented soy food, but it tastes and feels different. FoodData Central reports that tempeh has 7.64 grammes of carbohydrates and 20.3 grammes of protein per 100 grammes.

EDAMAME

With 11.9 grams of protein and 8.91 grams of carbohydrates in a 100-gram meal, edamame is comparatively high-protein and low-carb for a plant food. However, its macro ratios are more striking than those of tofu and tempeh.

ALMONDS

Almonds in their whole, uncooked form contain roughly 21 grams of protein for every 100 grams. Twenty-five grams of almonds, or around five grams of protein and five grams of carbohydrates, is a more reasonable serving size.

PUMPKIN SEEDS

Pumpkin seeds contain 10.7 grams of carbohydrates and 30.2 grams of protein per 100 grams. A one-ounce (28-gram) meal contains just 3 grams of carbohydrates and 8.6 grams of protein.

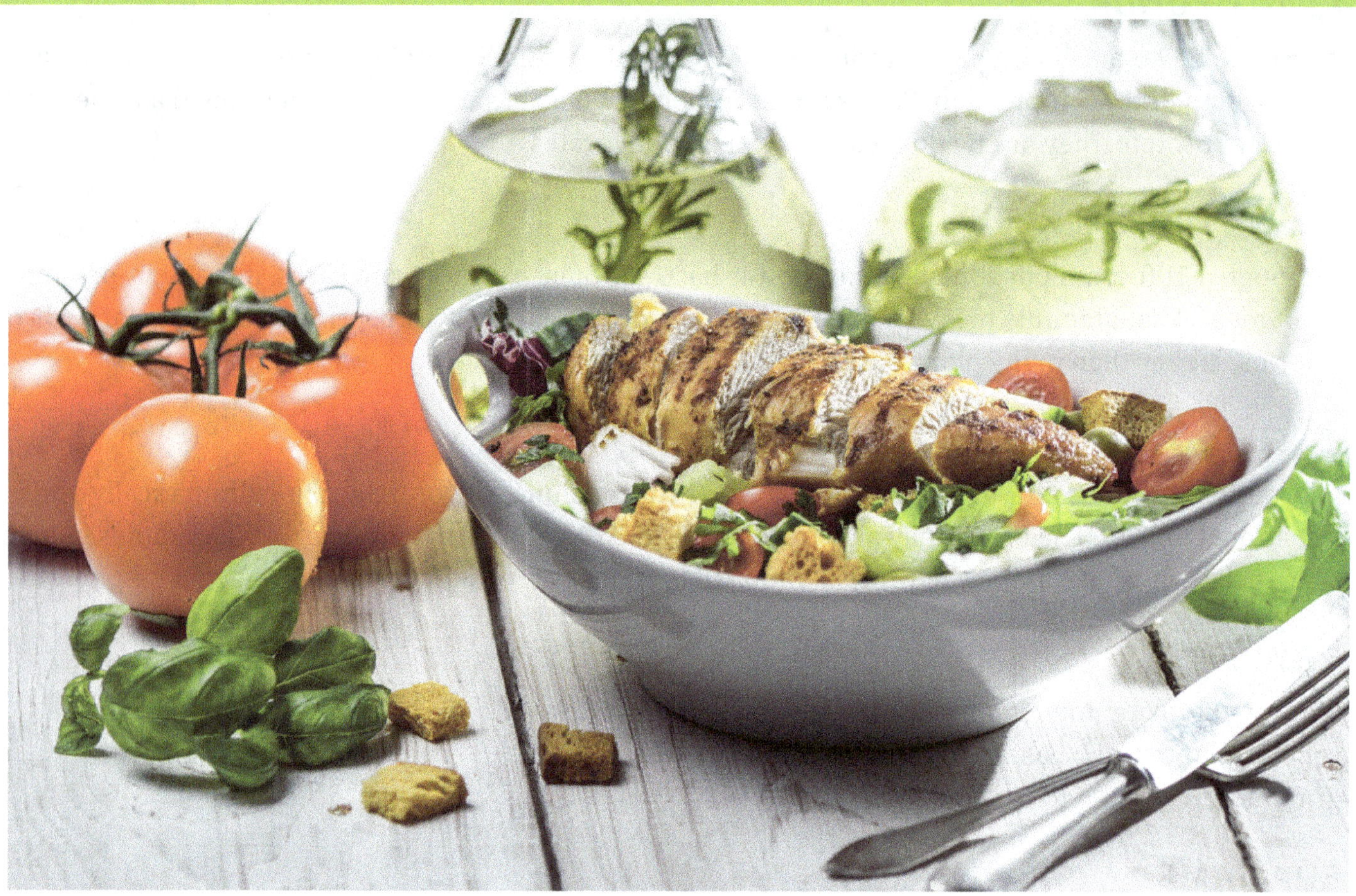

The possible health benefits have made a high-protein, low-carb diet increasingly fashionable. This book highlights the various ways that following this food plan may enhance many facets of one's health.

Controlling Weight and Reducing Fat:

This diet is favoured among so many people mainly because it works so well to control weight. Higher protein consumption is linked to higher satiety and a more substantial thermic impact because the body takes more energy to break down and digest proteins than fats or carbohydrates. In general, this leads to fewer calories consumed and promotes weight reduction. Moreover, it is essential to preserve muscle mass when losing weight and eating a lot of protein might help to maintain lean muscle mass.

Improved Blood Sugar Control:

People with diabetes or insulin resistance may find that a diet high in protein and low in carbs helps. Cutting less on carbs helps to steady blood sugar levels, which lessens the chance of swings in blood sugar after heavy meals. This diet may help improve general glycemic management since it reduces blood sugar rises and increases insulin sensitivity.

Enhanced Metabolic Health:

Many metabolic health indicators might be gained from this kind of eating. Research indicates that it may increase heart-healthy parameters such as HDL cholesterol, "good" cholesterol, and triglyceride levels. Furthermore, a diet heavy in protein and low in carbohydrates may lower blood pressure, essential for cardiovascular health.

Increased Muscle Mass and Strength:

As the building block of muscles, eating more protein may help with muscle development and repair, especially when accompanied by resistance training or other forms of exercise. Those who strength train may find this diet helpful since it promotes muscle repair and general strength gains.

Enhanced Satiety and Reduced Cravings:

Eating meals rich in protein has been demonstrated to enhance sensations of fullness and satisfaction. More protein will keep you fuller longer, which might lessen your desire to overindulge in high-calorie, unhealthy snacks or meals.

Taking Into Account Individual Variability:

It's crucial to consider personal differences even if a low-carb, high-protein diet has apparent benefits. This diet plan functions differently for each person. Depending on things like metabolic rate, degree of activity, and personal health problems, this diet may or may not benefit weight loss or overall health benefits.

A diet heavy in protein and light in carbohydrates has several benefits, such as increased muscle building, weight management, better blood sugar control, and better metabolic health. Finding a balance, receiving adequate nutrients, and considering your needs and preferences are all important aspects of any diet plan.

Find out about the advantages of this diet and adjust it to suit your lifestyle to take advantage of its potential to improve your overall health and wellness. Talking to a doctor or a qualified nutritionist before making significant dietary changes will help ensure that they align with your health goals and address any particular issues.

EGG-CELLENT VEGGIE SCRAMBLE

PREP TIME: 10 MINUTES | COOK TIME: 10 MINUTES
TOTAL TIME: 20 MINUTES

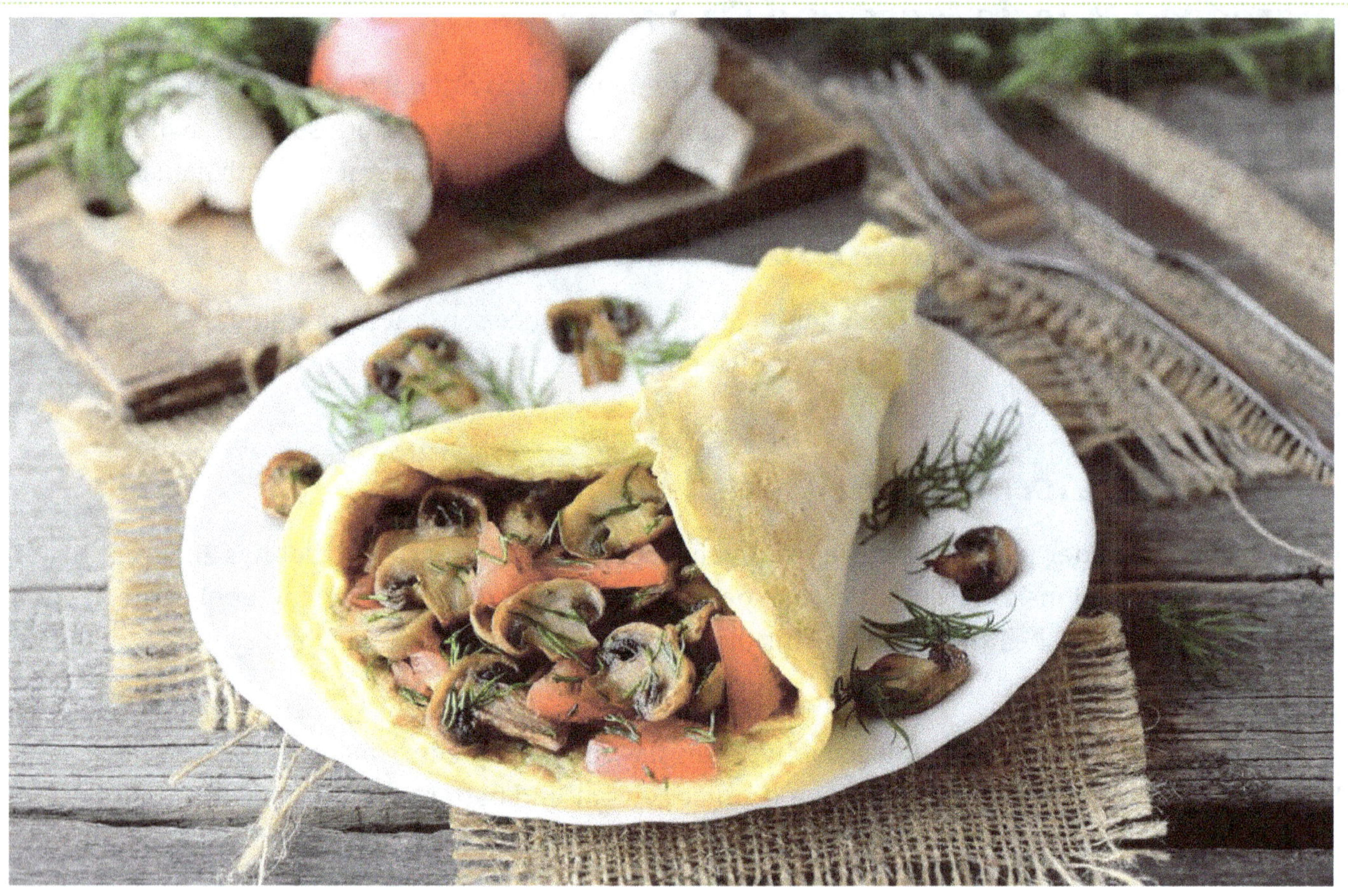

INGREDIENTS:

- 4 large eggs
- 1/2 cup diced bell peppers (any colour)
- 1/4 cup diced onions
- 1/4 cup diced tomatoes
- 1/4 cup chopped spinach
- Salt and pepper to taste
- 1 tablespoon olive oil

INSTRUCTIONS:

1. Whisk the eggs in a bowl and add pepper and salt to taste.
2. In a pan over medium heat, warm the olive oil.
3. When the onions and bell peppers are tender, add them and sauté.
4. Simmer the spinach and tomatoes for a further two minutes.
5. Add the whisked eggs and mix gradually until fully cooked.
6. Warm up the food.

NUTRITIONAL INFORMATION:
(PER SERVING)
CALORIES: 180
FAT: 12G
CARBOHYDRATES: 7G
PROTEIN: 12G

AVOCADO DELIGHT BREAKFAST BOWL

PREP TIME: 5 MINUTES | COOK TIME: 0 MINUTES
TOTAL TIME: 5 MINUTES

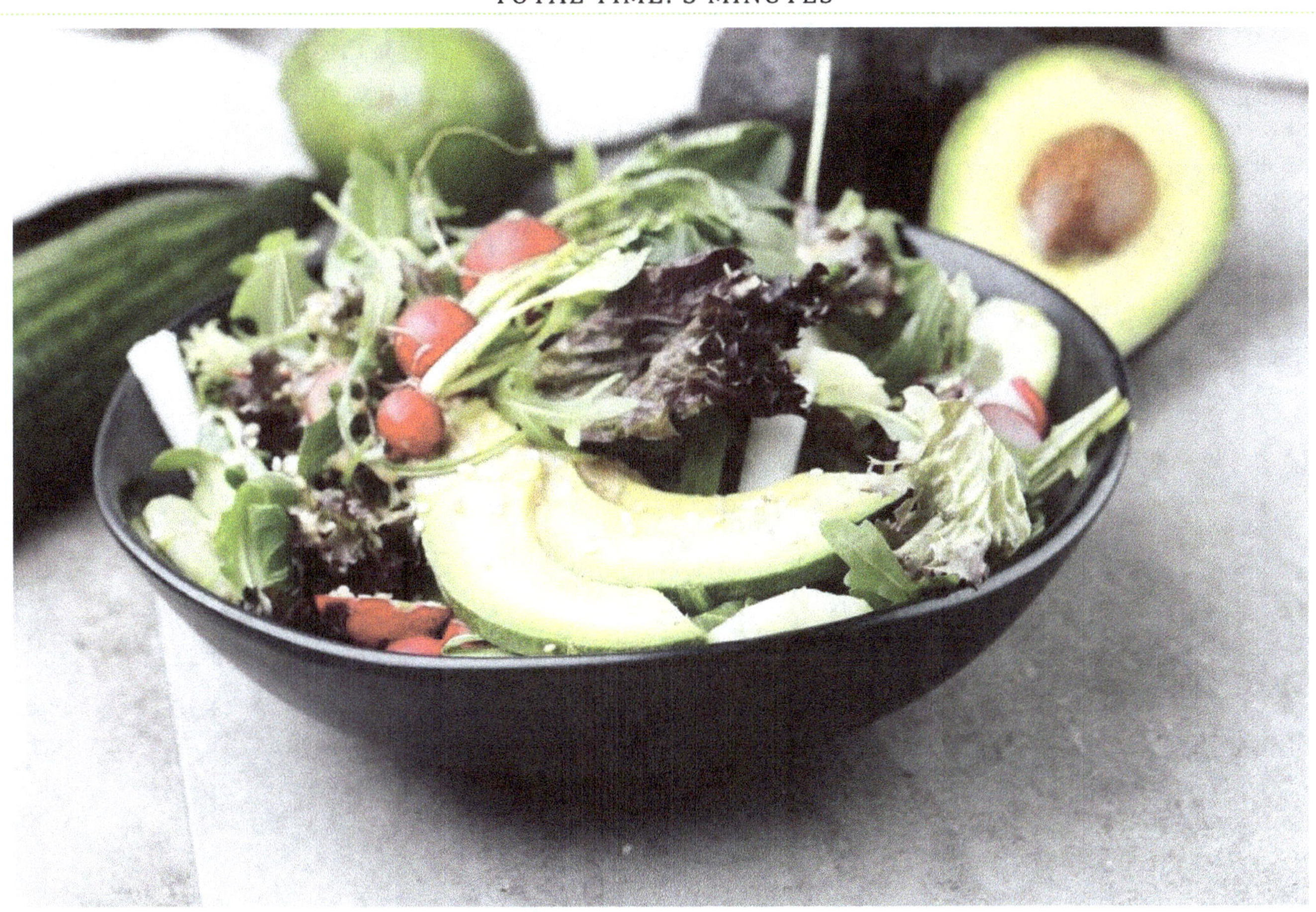

INGREDIENTS:
- 1 ripe avocado
- 2 eggs, boiled and sliced
- 1/2 cup cherry tomatoes, halved
- 1/4 cup crumbled feta cheese
- Salt and pepper to taste
- A drizzle of olive oil
- Fresh basil leaves for garnish

INSTRUCTIONS:
1. Halve the avocado and scoop out the pit.
2. Remove a small amount of flesh from each side to make more room for the filling.
3. Place the cherry tomatoes and pieces of cooked egg within the avocado halves.

4. Add salt and pepper for seasoning and pour over some olive oil.
5. Add some crumbled feta cheese on top, and some fresh basil leaves as a garnish.
6. Serve right away.

NUTRITIONAL INFORMATION:

(PER SERVING)
CALORIES: 320
FAT: 25G
CARBOHYDRATES: 12G
PROTEIN: 14G

BACON & SPINACH OMELETTE ROLL

PREP TIME: 5 MINUTES | COOK TIME: 10 MINUTES
TOTAL TIME: 15 MINUTES

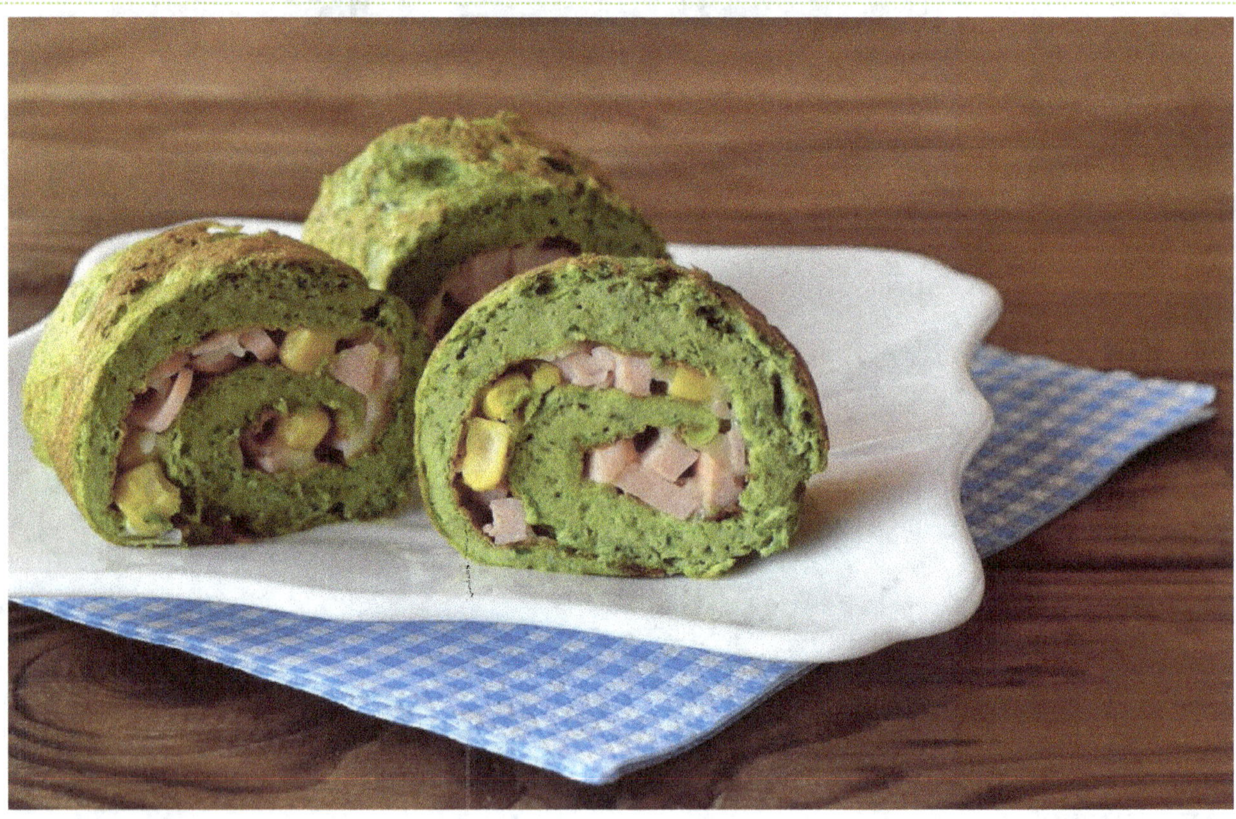

INGREDIENTS:

- 4 eggs
- 4 slices of bacon
- 1 cup fresh spinach leaves
- Salt and pepper to taste
- 1 tablespoon butter

INSTRUCTIONS:

1. Cut them into small pieces after crisping up bacon slices in a pan.
2. Beat the eggs and add salt and pepper to taste in a bowl.
3. In a nonstick pan, melt butter over medium heat.

4. After adding the beaten eggs to the pan, cook for a minute.
5. Top the omelette with chopped bacon and spinach leaves.
6. From one end to the other, carefully roll the omelette.
7. Take out of the pan and cut into serving sizes.
8. Warm up the food.

NUTRITIONAL INFORMATION:

(PER SERVING)
CALORIES: 280
FAT: 22G
CARBOHYDRATES: 1G
PROTEIN: 18G

KETO CAULIFLOWER HASH BROWNS

PREP TIME: 15 MINUTES | COOK TIME: 15 MINUTES
TOTAL TIME: 30 MINUTES

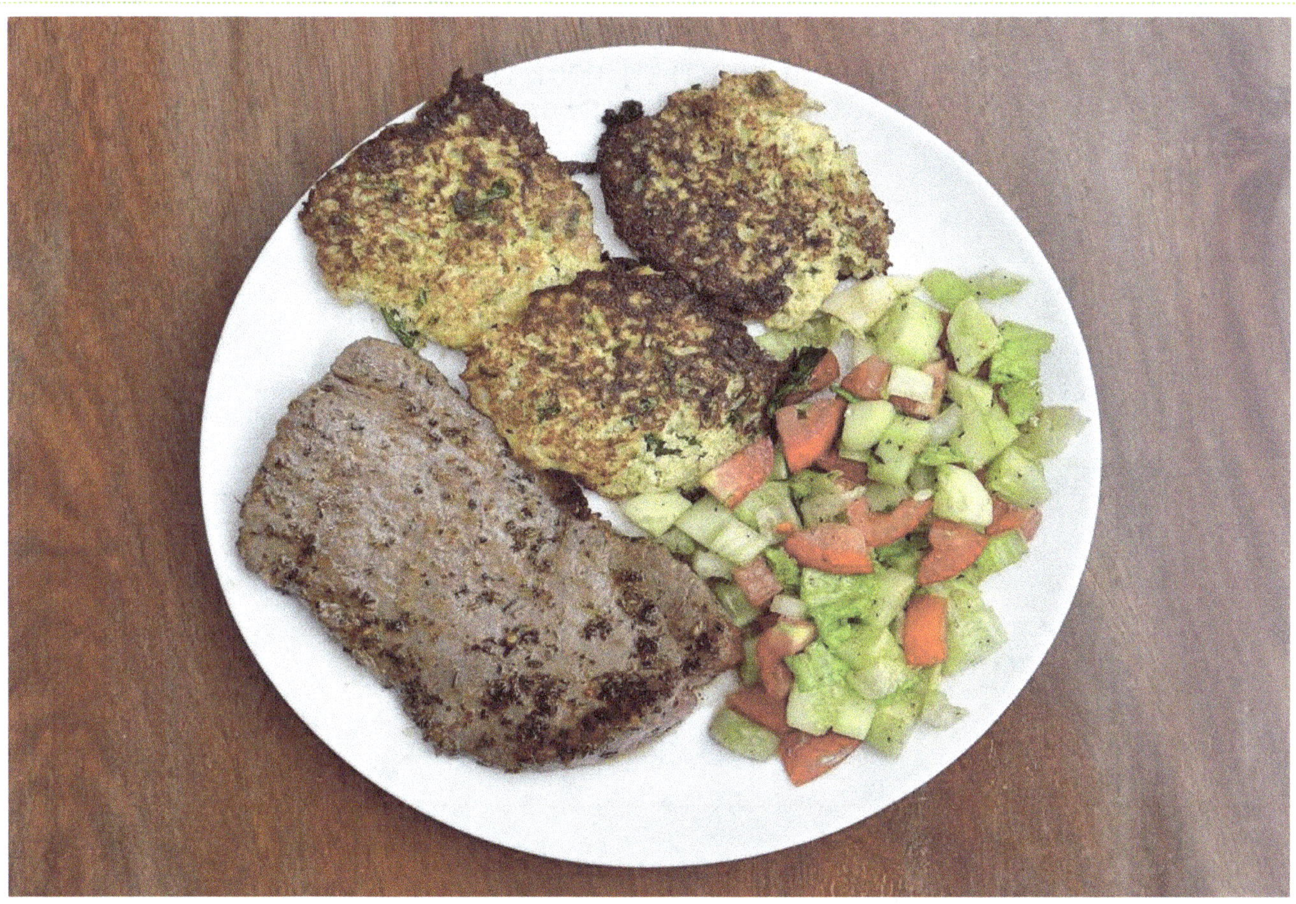

INGREDIENTS:

- 2 cups grated cauliflower
- 1/4 cup grated parmesan cheese
- 1/4 cup almond flour
- 2 eggs
- Salt and pepper to taste
- Cooking spray or olive oil for frying

INSTRUCTIONS:

1. Combine the grated cauliflower, eggs, almond flour, and parmesan cheese in a bowl.
2. Add salt and pepper for seasoning, then stir until well mixed.
3. Grease a skillet with cooking spray or a little olive oil and heat it over medium heat.
4. Form tiny patties by scooping the cauliflower mixture onto the grill.
5. Cook till golden brown, 3–4 minutes on each side.
6. Take out of the skillet and pat dry with paper towels.
7. Serve hot as an appetizer or for breakfast.

NUTRITIONAL INFORMATION:

(PER SERVING, 4 SERVINGS TOTAL)
CALORIES: 120
FAT: 8G
CARBOHYDRATES: 6G
PROTEIN: 8G

SMOKED SALMON & CREAM CHEESE WRAPS

PREP TIME: 10 MINUTES | COOK TIME: 0 MINUTES
TOTAL TIME: 10 MINUTES

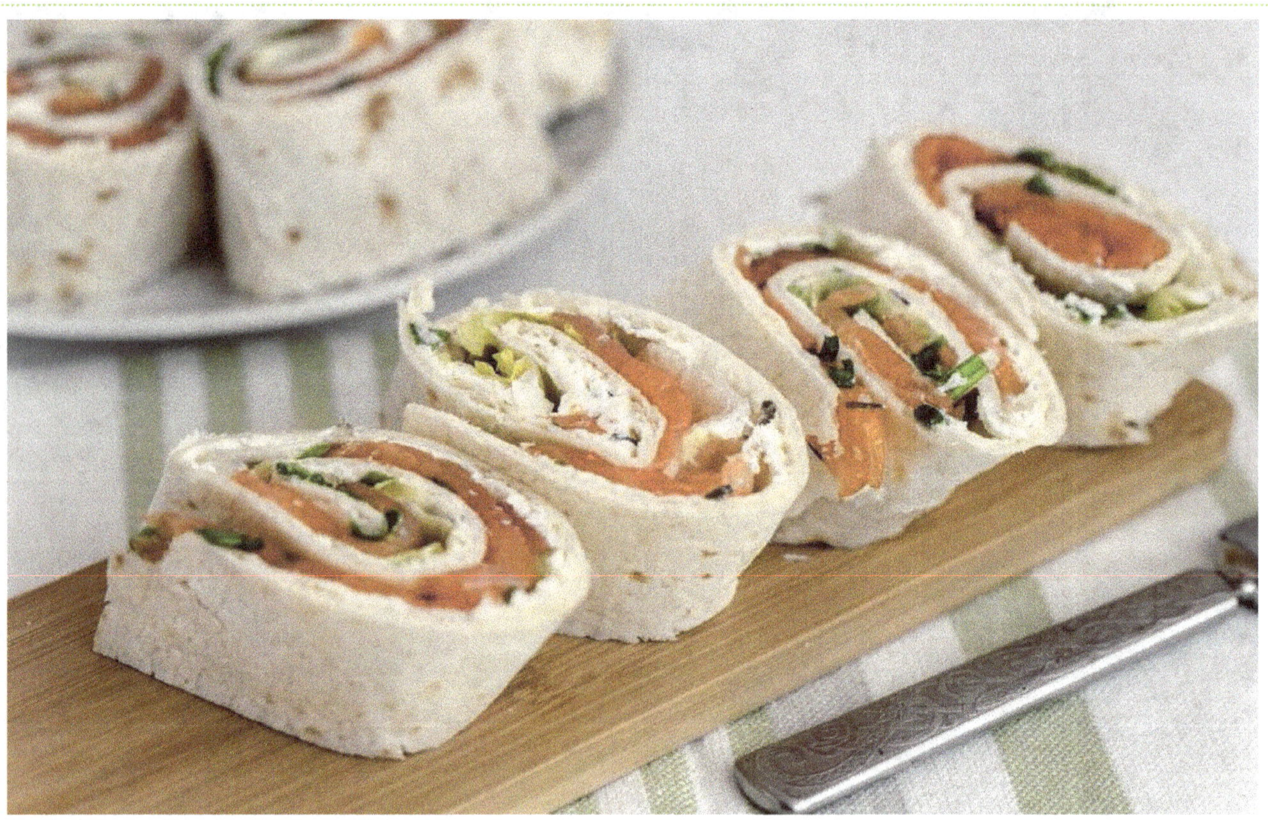

INGREDIENTS:

- 4 sizeable smoked salmon slices
- 1/2 cup cream cheese
- 1/4 cup diced cucumber
- 1/4 cup diced red onion
- 2 tablespoons capers

- Juice of 1/2 lemon
- Salt and pepper to taste
- 4 large lettuce leaves

INSTRUCTIONS:

1. Combine cream cheese, capers, lemon juice, sliced red onion, cucumber, and salt and pepper in a bowl.
2. Arrange the lettuce leaves on a spotlessly tidy tabletop.
3. Apply a coating of the cream cheese mixture to every leaf of lettuce.
4. Place a smoked salmon slice on top of the mixture of cream cheese.
5. To make lettuce wraps, carefully roll up the leaves.
6. Serve immediately or put in the fridge until you're ready to eat.

NUTRITIONAL INFORMATION:

(PER SERVING, 4 SERVINGS TOTAL)
CALORIES: 180
FAT: 12G
CARBOHYDRATES: 4G
PROTEIN: 14G

ZUCCHINI FRITTERS WITH SOUR CREAM DIP

PREP TIME: 15 MINUTES | COOK TIME: 15 MINUTES
TOTAL TIME: 30 MINUTES

INGREDIENTS:

- 2 medium zucchinis, grated
- 1/4 cup grated Parmesan cheese
- 1/4 cup almond flour
- 1 egg, beaten
- 2 cloves garlic, minced
- 2 tablespoons chopped fresh parsley
- Salt and pepper to taste
- Olive oil for frying

FOR SOUR CREAM DIP:

- 1/2 cup sour cream
- 1 tablespoon lemon juice
- 1 tablespoon chopped chives
- Salt and pepper to taste

INSTRUCTIONS:

1. Grated zucchini should be squeezed dry with a fresh kitchen towel.
2. Squeezed zucchini, Parmesan cheese, almond flour, beaten egg, minced garlic, chopped parsley, salt, and pepper should all be combined in a bowl.
3. In a pan over medium heat, warm the olive oil.
4. Flatten spoonfuls of the zucchini mixture using a spatula after adding them to the pan.
5. Cook till golden brown, 3–4 minutes on each side.
6. Transfer the cakes to a dish covered with paper towels to drain extra oil.

7. In a separate bowl, combine sour cream, lemon juice, chopped chives, salt, and pepper to make the sour cream dip.
8. Serve the hot zucchini fritters with a side of sour cream dip.

NUTRITIONAL INFORMATION:
(PER SERVING, WITHOUT DIP, 4 SERVINGS TOTAL)
CALORIES: 120
FAT: 8G
CARBOHYDRATES: 6G
PROTEIN: 6G

ALMOND FLOUR PANCAKES WITH BERRIES
PREP TIME: 10 MINUTES | COOK TIME: 10 MINUTES
TOTAL TIME: 20 MINUTES

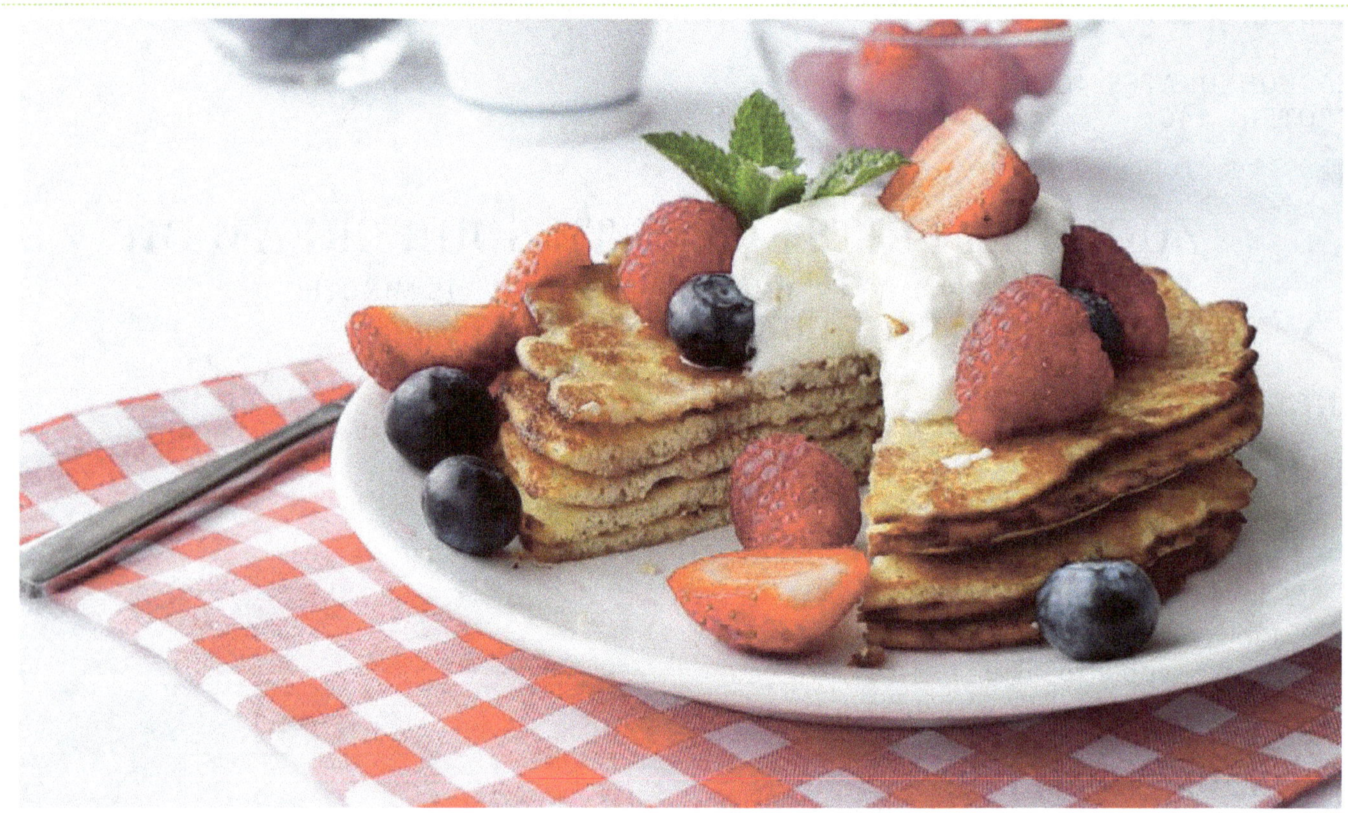

INGREDIENTS:
- 1 cup almond flour
- 2 large eggs
- 1/4 cup unsweetened almond milk
- 1 tablespoon coconut oil, melted
- 1 tablespoon honey or sweetener of choice (optional)
- 1 teaspoon baking powder
- 1/2 teaspoon vanilla extract
- Pinch of salt
- Fresh berries for topping
- Maple syrup for serving (optional)

INSTRUCTIONS:

1. Almond flour, eggs, almond milk, baking powder, vanilla extract, melted coconut oil, honey (if used), and salt should all be combined and whisked until smooth.
2. Grease a non-stick skillet or griddle with coconut oil and heat it over medium heat.
3. For each pancake, add about 1/4 cup of batter to the skillet.
4. Cook until golden brown, 2 to 3 minutes each side.
5. Proceed with the leftover batter.
6. If preferred, top pancakes with fresh berries and maple syrup before serving.

NUTRITIONAL INFORMATION:

(PER SERVING, WITHOUT TOPPINGS, 4 SERVINGS TOTAL)
CALORIES: 250
FAT: 20G
CARBOHYDRATES: 8G
PROTEIN: 10G

MEDITERRANEAN EGG MUFFINS

PREP TIME: 10 MINUTES | COOK TIME: 20 MINUTES
TOTAL TIME: 30 MINUTES

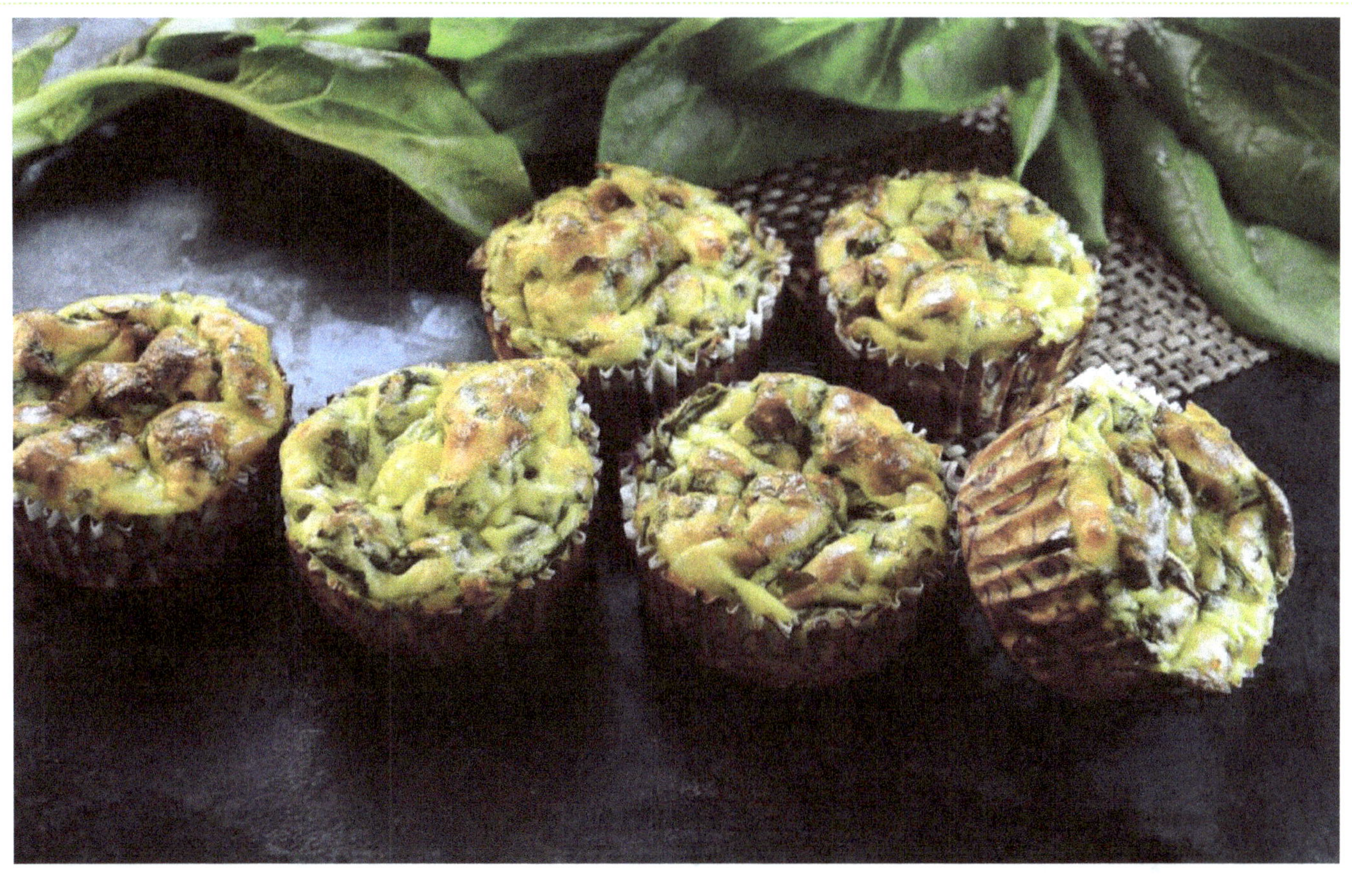

INGREDIENTS:

- 6 large eggs
- 1/4 cup diced bell peppers (any colour)
- 1/4 cup diced tomatoes
- 1/4 cup chopped spinach

- 1/4 cup crumbled feta cheese
- 1 tablespoon chopped fresh parsley
- Salt and pepper to taste
- Cooking spray or olive oil for greasing muffin tin

INSTRUCTIONS:

1. Set the oven's temperature to 175°C/350°F. Use olive oil or cooking spray to grease a muffin pan.
2. Whisk the eggs in a bowl and add pepper and salt to taste.
3. Add chopped parsley, crumbled feta cheese, diced tomatoes, bell peppers, and spinach.
4. Evenly fill the muffin tray with the egg mixture.
5. Bake the egg muffins for 18 to 20 minutes, or until they are set and have a hint of golden colour on top.
6. Before taking the egg muffins out of the muffin pan, let them cool somewhat.
7. Heat or serve at room temperature.

NUTRITIONAL INFORMATION:

(PER SERVING, 6 SERVINGS TOTAL)
CALORIES: 110
FAT: 7G
CARBOHYDRATES: 3G
PROTEIN: 9G

CHIA SEED PUDDING PARFAIT

PREP TIME: 5 MINUTES (PLUS CHILLING TIME) | COOK TIME: 0 MINUTES
TOTAL TIME: 5 MINUTES (PLUS CHILLING TIME)

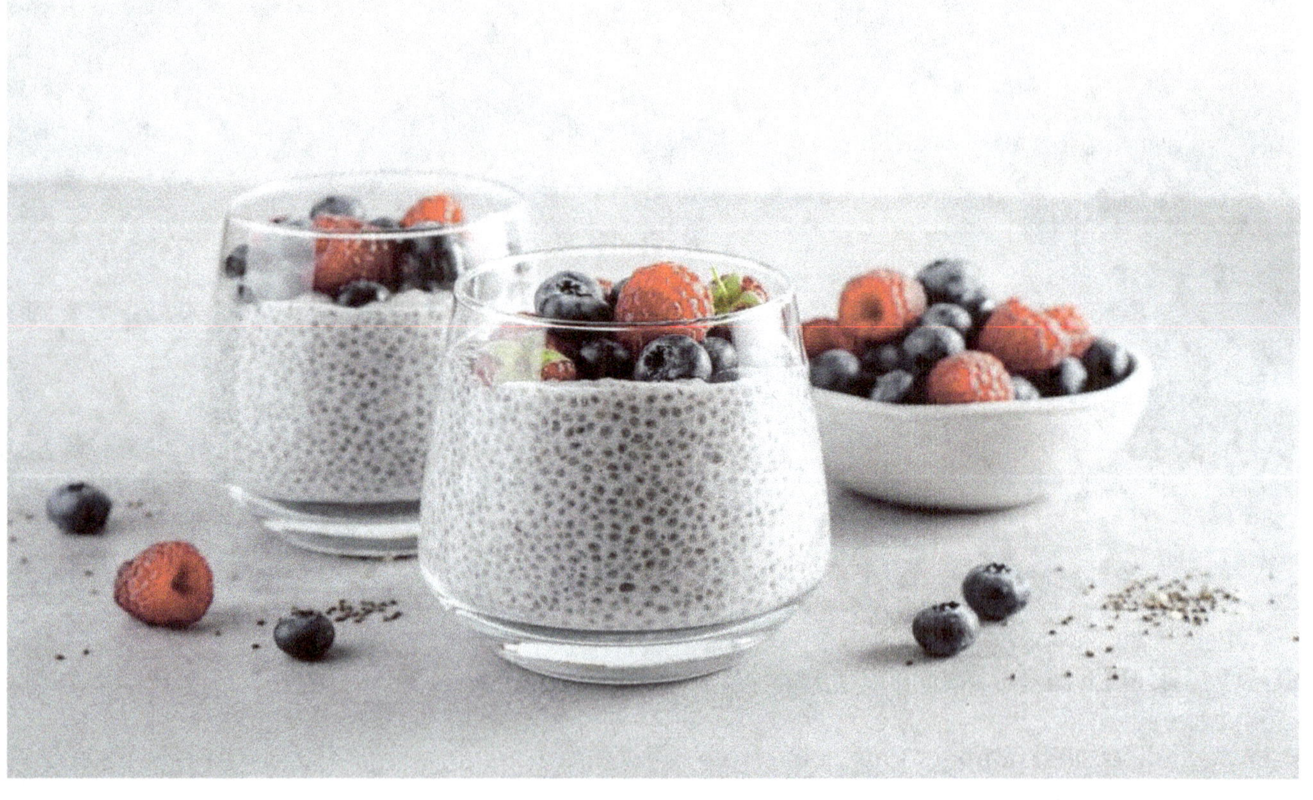

INGREDIENTS:

- 1/4 cup chia seeds
- 1 cup unsweetened almond milk
- 1 tablespoon honey or maple syrup (optional)
- 1/2 teaspoon vanilla extract
- Fresh berries
- Greek yoghurt
- Granola (optional)

INSTRUCTIONS:

1. Combine the chia seeds, almond milk, vanilla extract, honey (if used), and maple syrup in a bowl.
2. Once the mixture has thickened and become the consistency of pudding, cover the bowl and refrigerate it for at least two hours or overnight.
3. Arrange the parfait by stacking Greek yoghurt, chia seed pudding, and fresh berries into serving glasses.
4. Layers should be repeated until the glasses are full.
5. Add granola on top if you'd like.
6. Present cold.

NUTRITIONAL INFORMATION:

(PER SERVING, 2 SERVINGS TOTAL)
CALORIES: 180
FAT: 9G
CARBOHYDRATES: 20G
PROTEIN: 6G

GREEK YOGURT BREAKFAST SMOOTHIE

PREP TIME: 5 MINUTES | COOK TIME: 0 MINUTES
TOTAL TIME: 5 MINUTES

INGREDIENTS:

- 1 cup Greek yogurt
- 1/2 cup unsweetened almond milk
- 1/2 cup frozen mixed berries
- 1 tablespoon honey or maple syrup (optional)
- 1/2 teaspoon vanilla extract

INSTRUCTIONS:

1. Greek yoghurt, almond milk, frozen mixed berries, vanilla extract, honey, or maple syrup (if used) should all be combined in a blender.
2. Blend till creamy and smooth.
3. After transferring the smoothie into glasses, serve it right away.

NUTRITIONAL INFORMATION:

(PER SERVING, 2 SERVINGS TOTAL)
CALORIES: 150
FAT: 3G
CARBOHYDRATES: 17G

PROTEIN: 15G

KETO COCONUT PORRIDGE
PREP TIME: 5 MINUTES | COOK TIME: 5 MINUTES
TOTAL TIME: 10 MINUTES

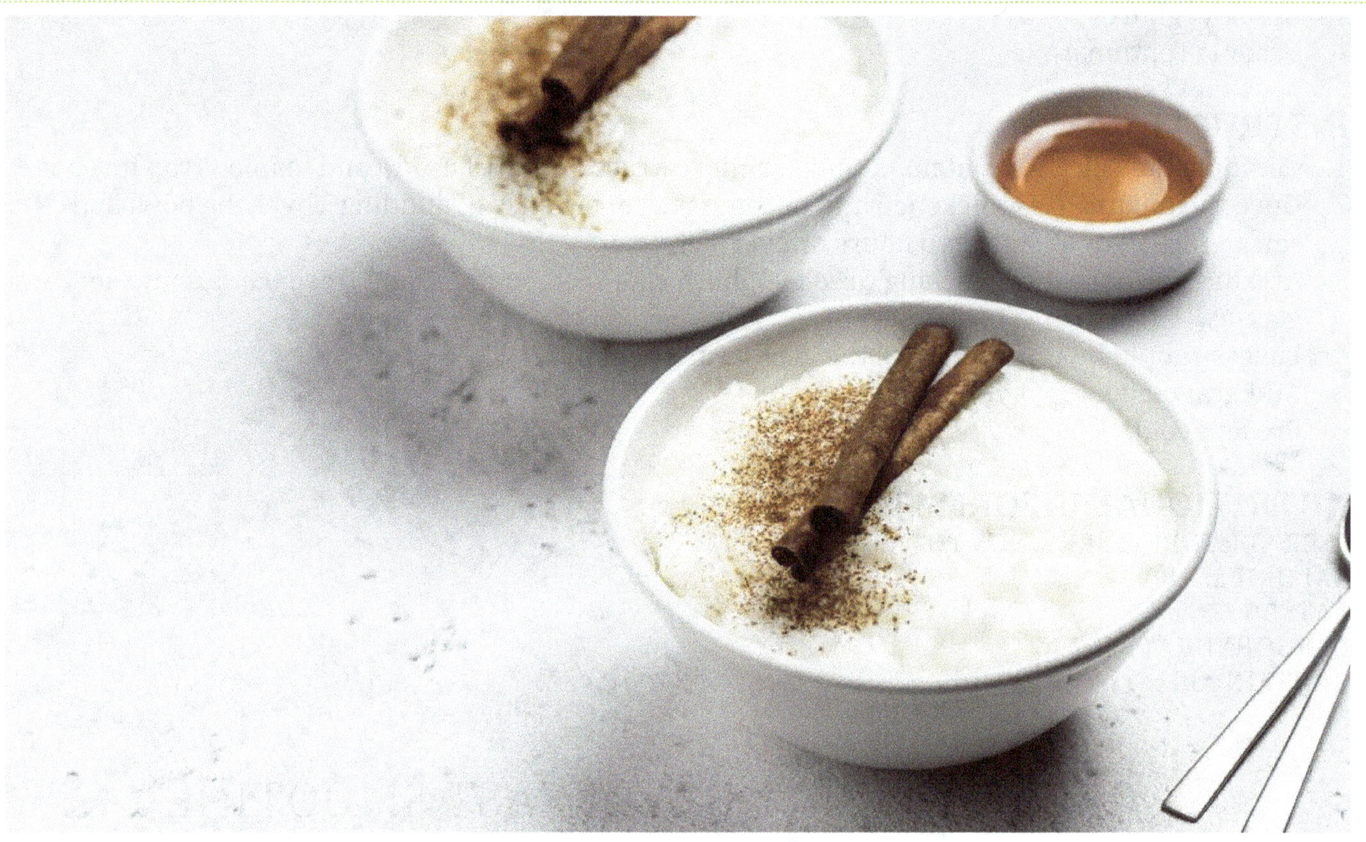

INGREDIENTS:
- 1/2 cup coconut flour
- 1 cup unsweetened coconut milk
- 1 tablespoon coconut oil
- 1 tablespoon chia seeds
- 1 tablespoon erythritol or sweetener of choice
- 1/4 teaspoon vanilla extract
- Pinch of salt
- Optional toppings: shredded coconut, sliced almonds, berries

INSTRUCTIONS:
1. Coconut flour, coconut milk, coconut oil, erythritol, chia seeds, vanilla essence, and a small salt should all be combined in a pot.
2. Stirring continuously, cook over medium heat until the porridge achieves the required consistency.
3. Take it off the stove and let it thicken for one minute.
4. Top with your preferred toppings and serve hot.

NUTRITIONAL INFORMATION:
(PER SERVING, 2 SERVINGS TOTAL)

CALORIES: 250
FAT: 18G
CARBOHYDRATES: 12G
FIBER: 8G
PROTEIN: 5G

TURKEY SAUSAGE BREAKFAST SKILLET

PREP TIME: 10 MINUTES | COOK TIME: 15 MINUTES
TOTAL TIME: 25 MINUTES

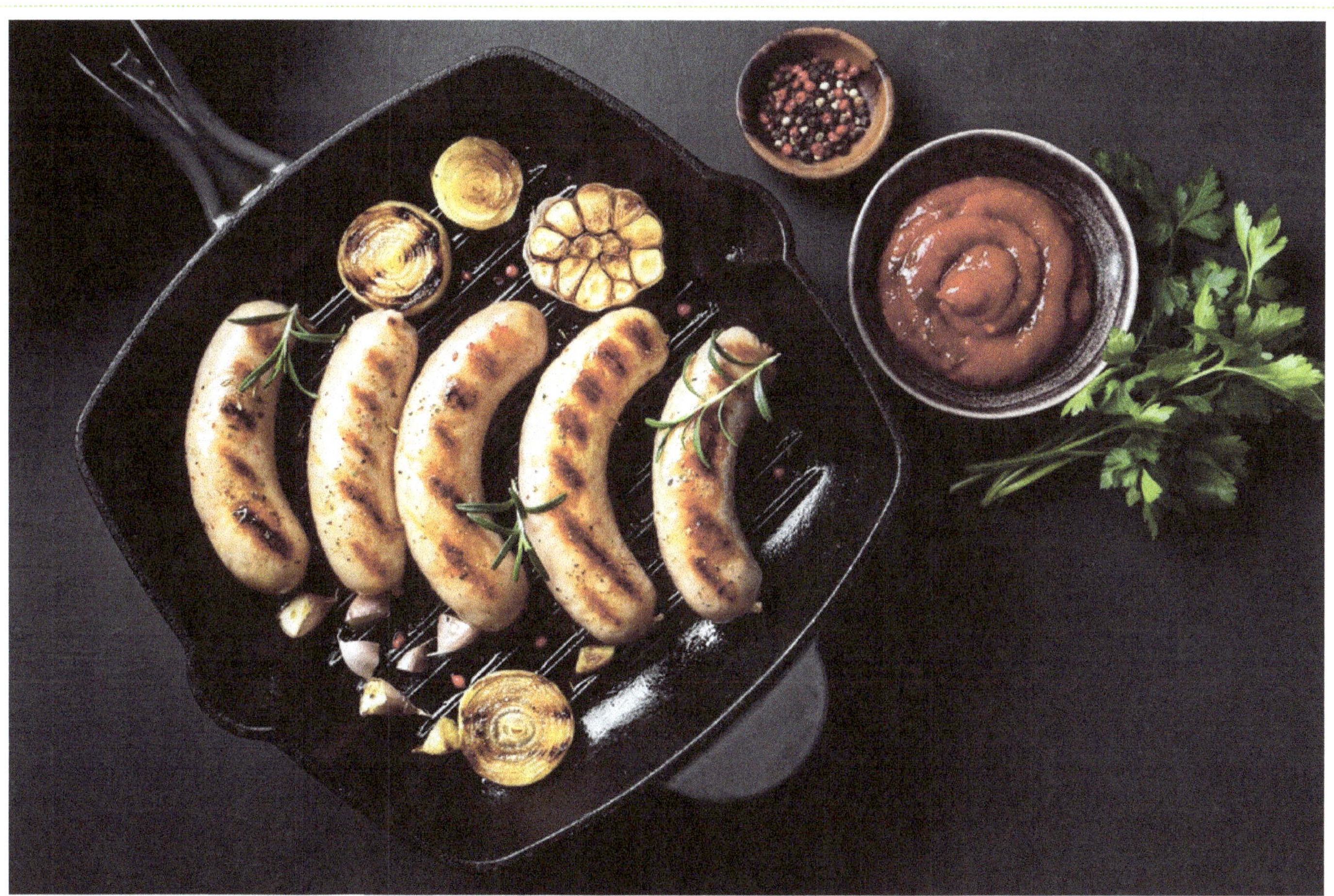

INGREDIENTS:

- 8 ounces turkey sausage, sliced
- 1 bell pepper, diced
- 1 small onion, diced
- 1 cup sliced mushrooms
- 4 eggs
- Salt and pepper to taste
- 1 tablespoon olive oil
- Fresh parsley for garnish (optional)

INSTRUCTIONS:

1. In a pan over medium heat, warm the olive oil.
2. Cook the turkey sausage pieces till they are browned.

3. Add chopped onion, bell pepper, and sliced mushrooms to the skillet.
4. Simmer until the sausage is done, and the veggies are tender.
5. Over the mixture, crack eggs and cook until done.
6. Add pepper and salt for seasoning.
7. If desired, garnish with fresh parsley.
8. Warm up the food.

NUTRITIONAL INFORMATION:

(PER SERVING, 2 SERVINGS TOTAL)
CALORIES: 320
FAT: 20G
CARBOHYDRATES: 10G
PROTEIN: 25G

CUCUMBER AND CREAM CHEESE SANDWICHES

PREP TIME: 10 MINUTES | COOK TIME: 0 MINUTES
TOTAL TIME: 10 MINUTES

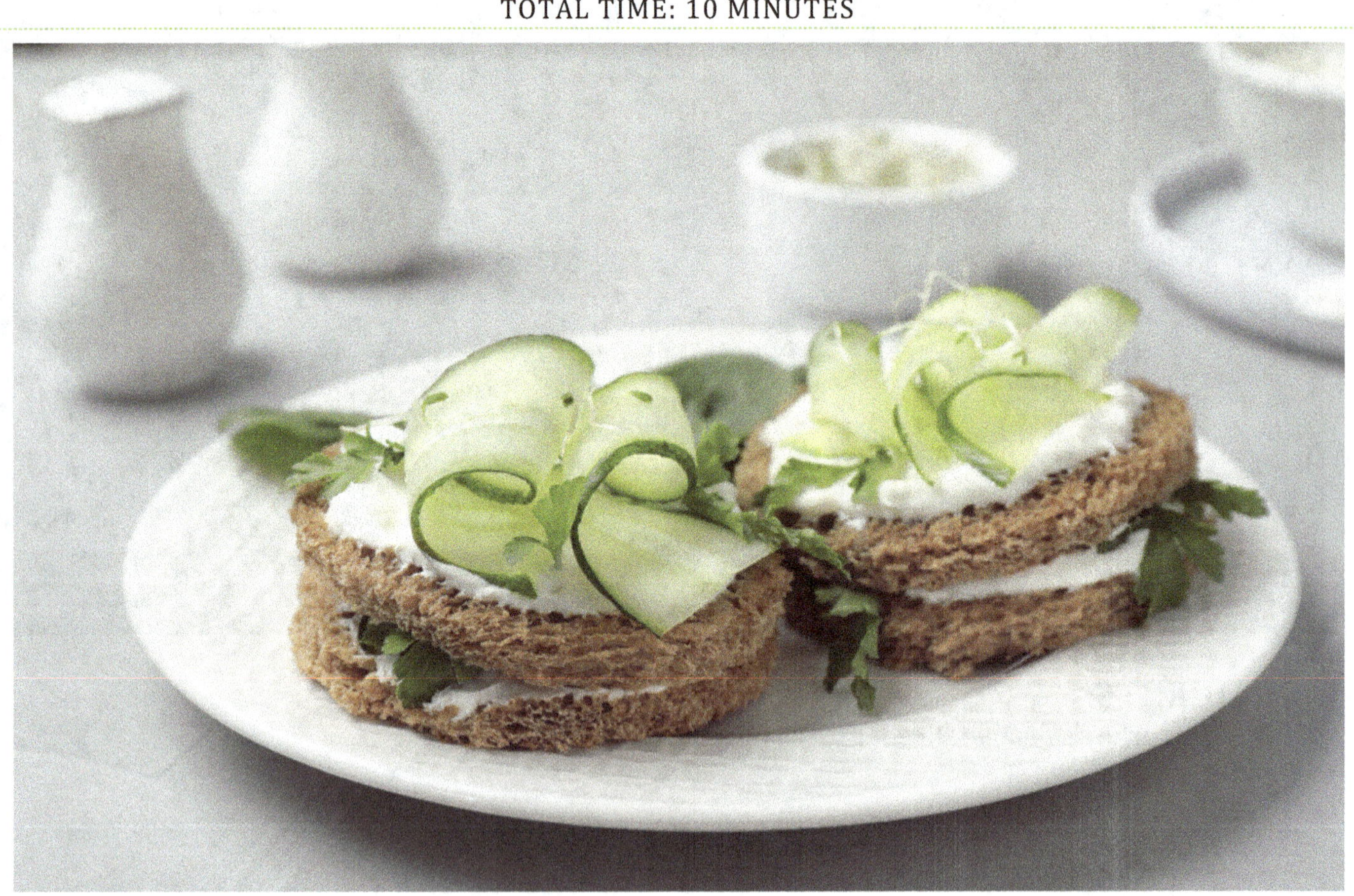

INGREDIENTS:

- 1 large cucumber, thinly sliced
- 1/2 cup cream cheese, softened
- 2 tablespoons chopped fresh dill
- Salt and pepper to taste
- Sliced bread of your choice (optional)

INSTRUCTIONS:

1. Combine melted cream cheese, chopped fresh dill, salt, and pepper in a bowl.
2. Drizzle a piece of bread (if using) with a layer of the cream cheese mixture.
3. Scatter the cucumber slices thinly over the cream cheese.
4. To assemble a sandwich, place another piece of bread on top (if using).
5. Continue using the remaining components.
6. If wanted, cut sandwiches into desired shapes.
7. Serve immediately or put in the fridge until you're ready to eat.

NUTRITIONAL INFORMATION:

(PER SERVING, 4 SERVINGS TOTAL, EXCLUDING BREAD)
CALORIES: 90
FAT: 8G
CARBOHYDRATES: 4G
PROTEIN: 2G

CAULIFLOWER CRUST QUICHE BITES

PREP TIME: 15 MINUTES | COOK TIME: 25 MINUTES
TOTAL TIME: 40 MINUTES

INGREDIENTS:

- 2 cups cauliflower rice
- 4 large eggs
- 1/4 cup milk or unsweetened almond milk
- 1/2 cup shredded cheddar cheese
- 1/4 cup diced bell peppers
- 1/4 cup diced onions
- Salt and pepper to taste
- Cooking spray

INSTRUCTIONS:

1. Turn the oven on to 375°F or 190°C. Grease a tiny muffin pan with cooking spray.
2. Microwave cauliflower rice for 3–4 minutes, or until it is tender, in a bowl that is safe to use in the microwave.
3. In a separate bowl, whisk together eggs, milk, shredded cheddar cheese, chopped onions, diced bell peppers, salt, and pepper.
4. Add the softened cauliflower rice and stir until well-mixed.
5. Fill each well to the brim of the small muffin tray by pouring the ingredients into it.
6. Bake the quiche bits for 20 to 25 minutes until they are set and have a light golden colour on top.
7. Before taking the quiche bits out of the muffin tray, let them cool somewhat.
8. Heat or serve at room temperature.

NUTRITIONAL INFORMATION:

(PER SERVING, 6 SERVINGS TOTAL)
CALORIES: 120
FAT: 8G
CARBOHYDRATES: 4G
PROTEIN: 8G

ALMOND BUTTER BANANA SMOOTHIE

PREP TIME: 5 MINUTES | COOK TIME: 0 MINUTES
TOTAL TIME: 5 MINUTES

INGREDIENTS:

- 1 ripe banana
- 2 tablespoons almond butter
- 1 cup unsweetened almond milk
- 1/2 teaspoon vanilla extract
- Optional: honey or maple syrup to sweeten

INSTRUCTIONS:

1. Put everything into a blender.
2. Blend till creamy and smooth.
3. For added sweetness, taste and add more honey or maple syrup as needed.
4. Transfer into glasses and serve right away.

NUTRITIONAL INFORMATION:

(PER SERVING, 2 SERVINGS TOTAL)
CALORIES: 230
FAT: 16G
CARBOHYDRATES: 19G
FIBER: 4G
PROTEIN: 6G

SPINACH AND MUSHROOM BREAKFAST CASSEROLE

PREP TIME: 15 MINUTES | COOK TIME: 35 MINUTES
TOTAL TIME: 50 MINUTES

INGREDIENTS:

- 8 large eggs
- 1 cup diced mushrooms
- 2 cups fresh spinach
- 1/2 cup diced onion
- 1/2 cup shredded cheddar cheese
- 1/4 cup milk or unsweetened almond milk
- Salt and pepper to taste
- Cooking spray or olive oil

INSTRUCTIONS:

1. Turn the oven on to 375°F, or 190°C. Use cooking spray or olive oil to grease a baking dish.
2. Diced mushrooms and onions should be softened by pan-frying them.
3. Cook the fresh spinach in the pan until it wilts.
4. Mix the eggs, milk, pepper, and salt in a bowl.
5. Evenly distribute the cooked veggies in the baking dish that has been prepared.
6. Cover the veggies with the egg mixture.
7. Top with shredded cheddar cheese.

8. Bake for thirty to thirty-five minutes or until the cheese is browned and the casserole is set.
9. Let the dish cool a little before cutting into slices and serving.

NUTRITIONAL INFORMATION:
(PER SERVING, 6 SERVINGS TOTAL)
CALORIES: 180
FAT: 12G
CARBOHYDRATES: 5G
PROTEIN: 13G

COCONUT FLOUR WAFFLES WITH WHIPPED CREAM
PREP TIME: 10 MINUTES | COOK TIME: 10 MINUTES
TOTAL TIME: 20 MINUTES

INGREDIENTS:
- 1/4 cup coconut flour
- 4 large eggs
- 1/4 cup coconut milk
- 2 tablespoons coconut oil, melted
- 1 tablespoon honey or sweetener of choice (optional)
- 1/2 teaspoon baking powder
- 1/2 teaspoon vanilla extract
- Pinch of salt
- Whipped cream for topping
- Fresh berries for topping

INSTRUCTIONS:
1. Warm up a waffle iron and spritz it with cooking spray or coconut oil.
2. To smooth the mixture, combine the coconut flour, eggs, coconut milk, melted coconut oil, baking powder, vanilla extract, and a small salt in a bowl. If using honey, whisk that in as well.
3. After pouring the batter onto the hot waffle iron, fry it as the maker directs until it becomes golden brown and crisps.
4. Present the warm waffles with whipped cream and fresh berries on top.

NUTRITIONAL INFORMATION:
(PER SERVING, 4 SERVINGS TOTAL)
CALORIES: 220
FAT: 16G
CARBOHYDRATES: 10G
FIBER: 3G
PROTEIN: 7G

LOW-CARB BREAKFAST BURRITO BOWL

PREP TIME: 10 MINUTES | COOK TIME: 15 MINUTES
TOTAL TIME: 25 MINUTES

INGREDIENTS:

- 4 large eggs
- 1 cup cauliflower rice
- 1/2 cup diced bell peppers
- 1/4 cup diced onions
- 1/4 cup shredded cheddar cheese
- 2 slices cooked bacon, chopped
- Salt and pepper to taste
- Avocado slices for topping
- Salsa for topping

INSTRUCTIONS:

1. Cook the eggs in a pan over medium heat until they are thoroughly done. Put aside.
2. Add the diced onions, bell peppers, and cauliflower rice to the same pan and cook until the ingredients are softened.
3. Add chopped cooked bacon, shredded cheddar cheese, and scrambled eggs to the pan. Stir until well hot and mixed.
4. To taste, add salt and pepper for seasoning.
5. Sort the mixture into separate dishes.
6. Before serving, garnish with avocado slices and salsa.

NUTRITIONAL INFORMATION:

(PER SERVING, 2 SERVINGS TOTAL)
CALORIES: 320
FAT: 22G
CARBOHYDRATES: 10G
FIBER: 4G
PROTEIN: 18G

BROCCOLI AND CHEESE EGG MUFFINS

PREP TIME: 10 MINUTES | COOK TIME: 20 MINUTES
TOTAL TIME: 30 MINUTES

INGREDIENTS:

- 6 large eggs
- 1 cup chopped broccoli florets
- 1/2 cup shredded cheddar cheese
- 1/4 cup diced onion
- Salt and pepper to taste
- Cooking spray

INSTRUCTIONS:

1. Turn the oven on to 375°F or 190°C. Grease a muffin tray with cooking spray.

2. Whisk the eggs, salt, and pepper in a bowl.
3. Add the sliced onion, shredded cheddar cheese, and chopped broccoli florets and stir until well-mixed.
4. Evenly transfer the mixture to the ready muffin tray.
5. Bake the egg muffins for 18 to 20 minutes until they are set and have a light golden colour on top.
6. Before taking the egg muffins out of the muffin pan, let them cool somewhat.
7. Heat or serve at room temperature.

NUTRITIONAL INFORMATION:

(PER SERVING, 6 SERVINGS TOTAL)
CALORIES: 120
FAT: 8G
CARBOHYDRATES: 3G
PROTEIN: 9G

PEANUT BUTTER PROTEIN BALLS

PREP TIME: 10 MINUTES | COOK TIME: 0 MINUTES
TOTAL TIME: 10 MINUTES

INGREDIENTS:

- 1 cup rolled oats
- 1/2 cup natural peanut butter
- 1/4 cup honey or maple syrup
- 1/4 cup protein powder (vanilla or chocolate)
- 1/4 cup mini chocolate chips (optional)
- 1 teaspoon vanilla extract

INSTRUCTIONS:

1. Blend the rolled oats, protein powder, honey, maple syrup, natural peanut butter, tiny chocolate chips (if used), and vanilla extract well in a bowl.
2. With your hands, roll the mixture into little balls.
3. Transfer the balls to a parchment paper-lined baking sheet.
4. To set, refrigerate for a minimum of half an hour.
5. The peanut butter protein balls should be in an airtight container in the refrigerator.

NUTRITIONAL INFORMATION:

(PER SERVING, ABOUT 10 SERVINGS TOTAL)
CALORIES: 150
FAT: 8G
CARBOHYDRATES: 15G
FIBER: 2G
PROTEIN: 7G

FLAXSEED ALMOND BREAD

PREP TIME: 10 MINUTES | COOK TIME: 40 MINUTES
TOTAL TIME: 50 MINUTES

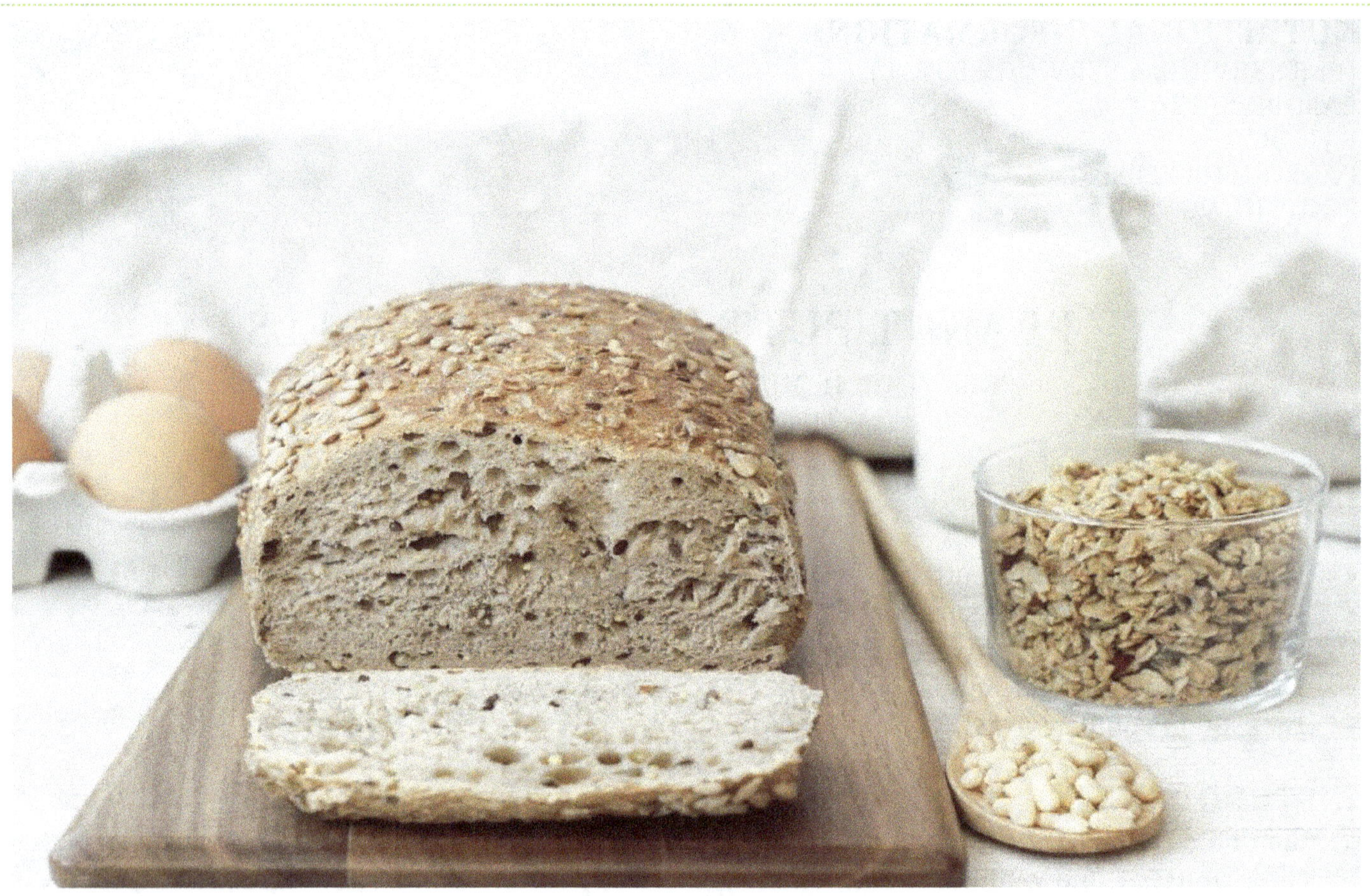

INGREDIENTS:

- 1 cup almond flour
- 1 cup ground flaxseed meal
- 1/4 cup coconut oil, melted
- 4 large eggs
- 1 teaspoon baking powder
- 1/2 teaspoon salt
- Optional: sesame seeds or poppy seeds for topping

INSTRUCTIONS:

1. Set the oven to 175°C/350°F. Grease or line a loaf pan with parchment paper with coconut oil.
2. Almond flour, powdered flaxseed meal, melted coconut oil, eggs, baking powder, and salt should all be mixed well in a big basin.
3. Using a spatula, level the top of the batter after it has been poured into the loaf pan.
4. If preferred, top with poppy or sesame seeds.
5. A toothpick put into the middle of the bread should come out clean after 35 to 40 minutes of baking or until the bread is golden brown.

6. Before slicing, let the bread sit in the pan for ten minutes and then move it to a wire rack to cool entirely.

NUTRITIONAL INFORMATION:
(PER SERVING, ABOUT 12 SERVINGS TOTAL)
CALORIES: 160
FAT: 14G
CARBOHYDRATES: 5G
FIBER: 4G
PROTEIN: 7G

COCONUT FLOUR ZUCCHINI BREAD
PREP TIME: 15 MINUTES | COOK TIME: 50 MINUTES
TOTAL TIME: 1 HOUR 5 MINUTES

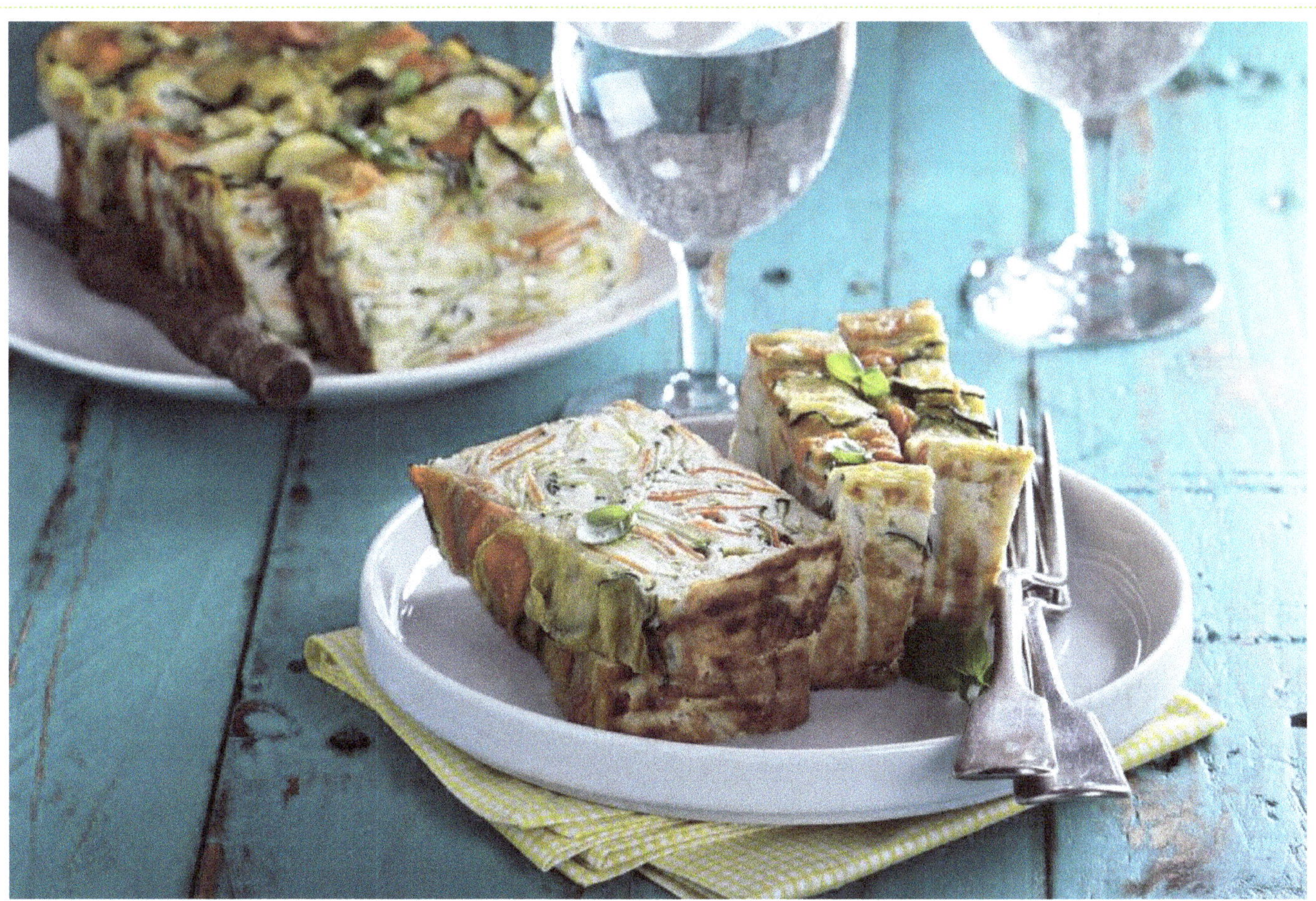

INGREDIENTS:
- 1 cup coconut flour
- 4 eggs
- 1/2 cup coconut oil, melted
- 1/4 cup honey or maple syrup
- 1 teaspoon baking powder
- 1 teaspoon ground cinnamon
- 1 teaspoon vanilla extract
- 1 cup grated zucchini

- Optional: chopped nuts or chocolate chips for topping

INSTRUCTIONS:

1. Set the oven to 175°C/350°F. Grease or line a loaf pan with parchment paper with coconut oil.
2. Coconut flour, eggs, melted coconut oil, honey, maple syrup, baking powder, cinnamon, and vanilla extract should all be combined in a big basin and whisked until smooth.
3. Grated zucchini should be included in the batter by folding it in evenly.
4. Transfer the mixture to the loaf pan that has been preheated and level it out.
5. If desired, top with chocolate chips or chopped nuts.
6. A toothpick put into the middle of the bread should come out clean after 45 to 50 minutes of baking or until the bread is golden brown.
7. Before slicing, let the bread sit in the pan for ten minutes and then move it to a wire rack to cool entirely.

NUTRITIONAL INFORMATION:
(PER SERVING, ABOUT 12 SERVINGS TOTAL)
CALORIES: 180
FAT: 12G
CARBOHYDRATES: 14G
FIBER: 5G
PROTEIN: 4G

KETO CLOUD BREAD ROLLS
PREP TIME: 15 MINUTES | COOK TIME: 25 MINUTES
TOTAL TIME: 40 MINUTES

INGREDIENTS:
- 3 large eggs, separated
- 3 tablespoons cream cheese, softened
- 1/4 teaspoon cream of tartar
- Pinch of salt

INSTRUCTIONS:

1. Set oven temperature to 300°F or 150°C. Use parchment paper to line a baking sheet.
2. Beat the egg whites and cream of tartar in a large bowl until firm peaks form.
3. In a separate basin, beat the egg yolks, melted cream cheese, and a little salt until smooth.
4. Till well blended, gently fold the egg yolk mixture into the beaten egg whites.
5. To create little cloud bread rolls, spoon batter onto the baking sheet that has been prepared.
6. Bake for 20 to 25 minutes, or until the tops of the cloud bread rolls are set and light golden in color.
7. Before serving, let the cloud bread rolls cool slightly.

NUTRITIONAL INFORMATION:
(PER SERVING, ABOUT 6 SERVINGS TOTAL)
CALORIES: 70
FAT: 5G
CARBOHYDRATES: 1G
PROTEIN: 4G

CHIA SEED PSYLLIUM HUSK BREAD

PREP TIME: 10 MINUTES | COOK TIME: 50 MINUTES
TOTAL TIME: 1 HOUR

INGREDIENTS:
- 1 cup almond flour
- 1/4 cup psyllium husk powder
- 1/4 cup chia seeds
- 4 large eggs
- 1/4 cup coconut oil, melted
- 1 teaspoon baking powder
- 1/2 teaspoon salt
- 1 tablespoon apple cider vinegar
- 1/4 cup water

INSTRUCTIONS:
1. Set the oven to 175°C/350°F. Grease or line a loaf pan with parchment paper with coconut oil.
2. Almond flour, chia seeds, psyllium husk powder, baking powder, and salt should all be combined in a big basin.
3. Whisk eggs, water, apple cider vinegar, and melted coconut oil in a separate basin.
4. After adding the wet components to the dry ingredients, thoroughly mix them.
5. Using a spatula to smooth the top, transfer the mixture into the loaf pan that has been prepped.
6. A toothpick put into the middle of the bread should come out clean after 45 to 50 minutes of baking or until the bread is golden brown.
7. Before slicing, let the bread sit in the pan for ten minutes and then move it to a wire rack to cool entirely.

NUTRITIONAL INFORMATION:
(PER SERVING, ABOUT 12 SERVINGS TOTAL)
CALORIES: 130
FAT: 10G
CARBOHYDRATES: 7G
FIBER: 5G
PROTEIN: 5G

LOW-CARB CAULIFLOWER BREADSTICKS

PREP TIME: 15 MINUTES | COOK TIME: 30 MINUTES
TOTAL TIME: 45 MINUTES

INGREDIENTS:
- 1 medium head cauliflower, grated
- 2 large eggs
- 1/2 cup shredded mozzarella cheese
- 1/4 cup grated Parmesan cheese
- 1 teaspoon Italian seasoning
- 1/2 teaspoon garlic powder
- Salt and pepper to taste

* Marinara sauce for dipping (optional)

INSTRUCTIONS:

1. Set the oven temperature to 425°F (220°C). Use parchment paper to line a baking sheet.
2. Grated cauliflower should be microwaved in a bowl designed for this purpose for 5 to 6 minutes, or until tender.
3. After letting the cauliflower cool, place it on a fresh kitchen towel and pat dry any remaining moisture.
4. Mix the cauliflower, eggs, grated Parmesan cheese, shredded mozzarella cheese, Italian seasoning, garlic powder, salt, and pepper in a big bowl. Blend until well blended.
5. Spread the cauliflower mixture evenly to create a rectangular shape on the baking sheet that has been prepared.
6. Bake for 25 to 30 minutes or until the breadsticks are firm and the edges are golden brown.
7. Before slicing the breadsticks into sticks, let them cool somewhat.
8. If preferred, serve with marinara sauce for dipping.

NUTRITIONAL INFORMATION:

(PER SERVING, ABOUT 6 SERVINGS TOTAL)
CALORIES: 90
FAT: 5G
CARBOHYDRATES: 5G
FIBER: 2G
PROTEIN: 7G

SESAME SEED KETO BREAD LOAF

PREP TIME: 15 MINUTES | COOK TIME: 50 MINUTES
TOTAL TIME: 1 HOUR 5 MINUTES

INGREDIENTS:

* 2 cups almond flour
* 1/4 cup coconut flour
* 1/4 cup ground flaxseed meal
* 1/4 cup sesame seeds
* 1 teaspoon baking powder
* 1/2 teaspoon baking soda
* 1/2 teaspoon salt
* 4 large eggs
* 1/4 cup melted coconut oil
* 1/4 cup unsweetened almond milk
* 1 tablespoon apple cider vinegar

INSTRUCTIONS:

1. Set the oven to 175°C/350°F. Grease or line a loaf pan with parchment paper with coconut oil.
2. Almond flour, coconut flour, sesame seeds, powdered flaxseed meal, baking powder, baking soda, and salt should all be combined in a big basin.
3. Beat the eggs in a separate basin. Mix well after adding the apple cider vinegar, almond milk, and melted coconut oil.
4. After adding the wet components to the dry ingredients, thoroughly mix them.

5. Using a spatula to smooth the top, transfer the mixture into the loaf pan that has been prepped.
6. If desired, sprinkle more sesame seeds on the top.
7. A toothpick put into the middle of the bread should come out clean after 45 to 50 minutes of baking or until the bread is golden brown.
8. Before slicing, let the bread sit in the pan for ten minutes and then move it to a wire rack to cool entirely.

NUTRITIONAL INFORMATION:
(PER SERVING, ABOUT 12 SERVINGS TOTAL)
CALORIES: 180
FAT: 15G
CARBOHYDRATES: 6G
FIBER: 3G
PROTEIN: 7G

CHEESE AND HERB KETO BISCUITS
PREP TIME: 10 MINUTES | COOK TIME: 15 MINUTES
TOTAL TIME: 25 MINUTES

INGREDIENTS:
- 2 cups almond flour
- 1/4 cup grated Parmesan cheese
- 2 teaspoons baking powder
- 1 teaspoon garlic powder
- 1 teaspoon dried Italian herbs
- 1/2 teaspoon salt
- 1/2 cup shredded cheddar cheese
- 2 large eggs
- 1/4 cup unsweetened almond milk
- 2 tablespoons melted butter

INSTRUCTIONS:
1. Set the oven's temperature to 175°C/350°F. Use parchment paper to line a baking sheet.
2. Almond flour, shredded cheddar cheese, baking powder, garlic powder, Italian herbs, and salt should all be combined in a big basin.
3. Beat the eggs in another basin. Add melted butter and almond milk and stir.
4. After adding the wet components to the dry ingredients, thoroughly mix them.
5. To create biscuits, scoop dough onto a baking sheet that has been prepared.
6. Bake the biscuits for 12 to 15 minutes or until they are cooked through and golden brown.
7. Before serving, let the biscuits cool somewhat.

NUTRITIONAL INFORMATION:
(PER SERVING, ABOUT 8 SERVINGS TOTAL)
CALORIES: 230
FAT: 19G
CARBOHYDRATES: 6G
FIBER: 3G
PROTEIN: 9G

ALMOND FLOUR ROSEMARY FOCACCIA

PREP TIME: 10 MINUTES | COOK TIME: 25 MINUTES
TOTAL TIME: 35 MINUTES

INGREDIENTS:
- 2 cups almond flour
- 1/4 cup olive oil
- 2 tablespoons fresh rosemary, chopped
- 1 teaspoon baking powder
- 1/2 teaspoon salt
- 2 large eggs
- 1/4 cup water
- Sea salt flakes for topping

INSTRUCTIONS:
1. Set the oven's temperature to 175°C/350°F. Use parchment paper to line a baking sheet.
2. In a large bowl, combine almond flour, baking powder, salt, olive oil, and freshly chopped rosemary.
3. Beat the eggs in another basin. Add water and stir.
4. After adding the wet components to the dry ingredients, thoroughly mix them.
5. After transferring the dough to the baking sheet that has been prepared, push it out evenly to make a rectangle.
6. Top the dough with flakes of sea salt.
7. Bake the focaccia for 20 to 25 minutes or until it is cooked through and golden brown.
8. Let cool somewhat before slicing and serving focaccia.

NUTRITIONAL INFORMATION:
(PER SERVING, ABOUT 8 SERVINGS TOTAL)
CALORIES: 220
FAT: 20G
CARBOHYDRATES: 6G
FIBER: 3G
PROTEIN: 7G

PUMPKIN SEED FLAX BREAD

PREP TIME: 15 MINUTES | COOK TIME: 50 MINUTES
TOTAL TIME: 1 HOUR 5 MINUTES

INGREDIENTS:
- 1 1/2 cups almond flour
- 1/2 cup ground flaxseed meal
- 1/4 cup pumpkin seeds
- 1 teaspoon baking powder
- 1/2 teaspoon baking soda
- 1/2 teaspoon salt
- 4 large eggs
- 1/4 cup melted coconut oil
- 1/4 cup unsweetened almond milk

- 1 tablespoon apple cider vinegar

INSTRUCTIONS:
1. Set the oven to 175°C/350°F. Grease or line a loaf pan with parchment paper with coconut oil.
2. Almond flour, pumpkin seeds, powdered flaxseed meal, baking powder, baking soda, and salt should all be combined in a big basin.
3. Beat the eggs in a separate basin. Mix well after adding the apple cider vinegar, almond milk, and melted coconut oil.
4. After adding the wet components to the dry ingredients, thoroughly mix them together.
5. Using a spatula to smooth the top, transfer the mixture into the loaf pan that has been prepped.
6. A toothpick put into the middle of the bread should come out clean after 45 to 50 minutes of baking or until the bread is golden brown.
7. Before slicing, let the bread sit in the pan for ten minutes and then move it to a wire rack to cool entirely.

NUTRITIONAL INFORMATION:
(PER SERVING, ABOUT 12 SERVINGS TOTAL)
CALORIES: 180
FAT: 15G
CARBOHYDRATES: 6G
FIBER: 3G
PROTEIN: 7G

SPINACH AND FETA CHEESE BREAD
PREP TIME: 15 MINUTES | COOK TIME: 50 MINUTES
TOTAL TIME: 1 HOUR 5 MINUTES

INGREDIENTS:
- 2 cups almond flour
- 1/4 cup coconut flour
- 1/4 cup grated Parmesan cheese
- 1 teaspoon baking powder
- 1/2 teaspoon baking soda
- 1/2 teaspoon salt
- 4 large eggs
- 1/4 cup melted butter
- 1/4 cup unsweetened almond milk
- 1 tablespoon apple cider vinegar
- 1 cup chopped fresh spinach
- 1/2 cup crumbled feta cheese

INSTRUCTIONS:
1. Set the oven to 175°C/350°F. Grease or line a loaf pan with parchment paper with coconut oil.
2. Combine the almond flour, coconut flour, grated Parmesan cheese, baking soda, baking powder, and salt in a big basin.
3. Beat the eggs in a separate basin. Mix well after adding the melted butter, almond milk, and apple cider vinegar.
4. After adding the wet components to the dry ingredients, thoroughly mix them together.

5. In order to spread the feta cheese crumbles and chopped fresh spinach equally throughout the batter, fold them in.
6. Using a spatula to smooth the top, transfer the mixture into the loaf pan that has been prepped.
7. A toothpick put into the middle of the bread should come out clean after 45 to 50 minutes of baking or until the bread is golden brown.
8. Before slicing, let the bread sit in the pan for ten minutes and then move it to a wire rack to cool entirely.

NUTRITIONAL INFORMATION:
(PER SERVING, ABOUT 12 SERVINGS TOTAL)
CALORIES: 190
FAT: 15G
CARBOHYDRATES: 6G
FIBER: 3G
PROTEIN: 7G

SUNFLOWER SEED KETO FLATBREAD
PREP TIME: 10 MINUTES | COOK TIME: 15 MINUTES
TOTAL TIME: 25 MINUTES

INGREDIENTS:
- 1 cup almond flour
- 1/4 cup ground flaxseed meal
- 1/4 cup sunflower seeds
- 1 teaspoon baking powder
- 1/2 teaspoon garlic powder
- 1/2 teaspoon dried Italian herbs
- 1/4 teaspoon salt
- 2 large eggs
- 1/4 cup water
- 2 tablespoons olive oil

INSTRUCTIONS:
1. Set the oven's temperature to 175°C/350°F. Use parchment paper to line a baking sheet.
2. Almond flour, ground flaxseed meal, sunflower seeds, baking powder, garlic powder, Italian herbs, and salt should all be combined in a big basin.
3. Beat the eggs in another basin. Add olive oil and water, and stir.
4. After adding the wet components to the dry ingredients, thoroughly mix them.
5. Press the dough uniformly to make a flatbread after transferring it to the baking sheet that has been prepared.
6. Bake the flatbread for 12 to 15 minutes or until it's cooked through and golden brown.
7. Let the flatbread cool a little before cutting it into slices and serving.

NUTRITIONAL INFORMATION:
(PER SERVING, ABOUT 6 SERVINGS TOTAL)
CALORIES: 190
FAT: 16G
CARBOHYDRATES: 6G

FIBER: 3G
PROTEIN: 7G

WALNUT FLOUR BANANA BREAD

PREP TIME: 15 MINUTES | COOK TIME: 50 MINUTES
TOTAL TIME: 1 HOUR 5 MINUTES

INGREDIENTS:
- 2 cups walnut flour
- 1 teaspoon baking powder
- 1/2 teaspoon baking soda
- 1/2 teaspoon ground cinnamon
- 1/4 teaspoon salt
- 2 large ripe bananas, mashed
- 1/4 cup melted coconut oil
- 1/4 cup honey or maple syrup
- 2 large eggs
- 1 teaspoon vanilla extract

INSTRUCTIONS:
1. Set the oven to 175°C/350°F. Grease or line a loaf pan with parchment paper with coconut oil.
2. Mix the walnut flour, baking soda, baking powder, cinnamon, and salt in a large basin.
3. Mash the bananas and thoroughly blend them with the melted coconut oil, eggs, vanilla extract, honey, or maple syrup in a separate dish.
4. Mixing until just mixed, pour the wet components into the dry ingredients.
5. Using a spatula to smooth the top, transfer the mixture into the loaf pan that has been prepped.
6. A toothpick put into the middle of the bread should come out clean after 45 to 50 minutes of baking or until the bread is golden brown.
7. Before slicing, let the bread sit in the pan for ten minutes and then move it to a wire rack to cool entirely.

NUTRITIONAL INFORMATION:
(PER SERVING, ABOUT 12 SERVINGS TOTAL)
CALORIES: 200
FAT: 16G
CARBOHYDRATES: 12G
FIBER: 2G
PROTEIN: 5G

CUCUMBER AND CREAM CHEESE BITES

PREP TIME: 15 MINUTES | COOK TIME: 0 MINUTES
TOTAL TIME: 15 MINUTES

INGREDIENTS:

- 1 large cucumber
- 4 oz cream cheese, softened
- 1 tablespoon fresh dill, chopped
- Salt and pepper to taste

INSTRUCTIONS:

1. After cleaning, cut the cucumber into rounds that are 1/4 inch thick.
2. Combine melted cream cheese, chopped fresh dill, salt, and pepper in a small bowl.
3. Apply a thin coating of the cream cheese mixture on each cucumber round.
4. Serve immediately or put in the fridge until you're ready to serve.

NUTRITIONAL INFORMATION:

(PER SERVING, ABOUT 4 SERVINGS TOTAL)
CALORIES: 90
FAT: 8G
CARBOHYDRATES: 3G
PROTEIN: 2G

BACON-WRAPPED ASPARAGUS SPEARS

PREP TIME: 10 MINUTES | COOK TIME: 20 MINUTES
TOTAL TIME: 30 MINUTES

INGREDIENTS:

- 1 bunch asparagus spears
- 8 slices bacon

INSTRUCTIONS:

1. Set oven temperature to 400°F, or 200°C. Use parchment paper to line a baking sheet.
2. Trim the asparagus stalks of their woody ends.
3. Asparagus spears should be divided into bundles of roughly four to five.
4. Starting from the bottom, wrap a piece of bacon around each bundle, encircling the spears.
5. Spread the bundles of asparagus with bacon on the baking sheet that has been preheated.
6. Bake for 15 to 20 minutes or until the asparagus is soft and the bacon is crispy.
7. Serve right away.

NUTRITIONAL INFORMATION:

(PER SERVING, ABOUT 4 SERVINGS TOTAL)
CALORIES: 150

FAT: 11G
CARBOHYDRATES: 2G
PROTEIN: 10G

KETO CAPRESE SKEWERS

PREP TIME: 15 MINUTES | COOK TIME: 0 MINUTES
TOTAL TIME: 15 MINUTES

INGREDIENTS:
- Cherry tomatoes
- Fresh mozzarella balls
- Fresh basil leaves
- Balsamic glaze (optional)
- Toothpicks or skewers

INSTRUCTIONS:
1. Thread one cherry tomato, one fresh mozzarella ball, and one fresh basil leaf on each toothpick or skewer.
2. Place the caprese skewers on a plate for serving.
3. If desired, drizzle with balsamic glaze.
4. Serve right away.

NUTRITIONAL INFORMATION:
(PER SERVING, ABOUT 4 SERVINGS TOTAL)
CALORIES: 70
FAT: 5G
CARBOHYDRATES: 2G
PROTEIN: 4G

AVOCADO STUFFED WITH TUNA SALAD

PREP TIME: 15 MINUTES | COOK TIME: 0 MINUTES
TOTAL TIME: 15 MINUTES

INGREDIENTS:
- 2 ripe avocados
- 1 can (5 oz) tuna, drained
- 2 tablespoons mayonnaise
- 1 tablespoon diced red onion
- 1 tablespoon diced celery
- 1 tablespoon chopped fresh parsley
- Salt and pepper to taste
- Lemon wedges for serving (optional)

INSTRUCTIONS:
1. Halve the avocados and scoop out the pits.

2. Combine the drained tuna, mayonnaise, celery, diced onion, chopped fresh parsley, salt, and pepper in a bowl.
3. Fill the avocado halves with the tuna salad.
4. If preferred, serve right away with lemon slices.

NUTRITIONAL INFORMATION:

(PER SERVING, ABOUT 4 SERVINGS TOTAL)
CALORIES: 220
FAT: 18G
CARBOHYDRATES: 6G
PROTEIN: 9G

ZUCCHINI PARMESAN CHIPS

PREP TIME: 10 MINUTES | COOK TIME: 20 MINUTES
TOTAL TIME: 30 MINUTES

INGREDIENTS:

- 2 medium zucchinis
- 1/2 cup grated Parmesan cheese
- 1/2 teaspoon garlic powder
- 1/2 teaspoon dried oregano
- Salt and pepper to taste
- Olive oil spray

INSTRUCTIONS:

1. Set the oven temperature to 425°F (220°C). Use parchment paper to line a baking sheet.
2. Cut the zucchinis into thin rounds—roughly 1/4 inch thick.
3. Combine the grated Parmesan cheese, dried oregano, garlic powder, salt, and pepper in a bowl.
4. Arrange the zucchini slices in a single layer on the baking sheet that has been prepared.
5. Apply a thin layer of olive oil spray to the zucchini slices.
6. Evenly distribute the Parmesan mixture over the pieces of zucchini.
7. Bake the zucchini chips for 15 to 20 minutes or until they are crispy and golden brown.
8. Before serving, allow the chips to cool somewhat.

NUTRITIONAL INFORMATION:

(PER SERVING, ABOUT 4 SERVINGS TOTAL)
CALORIES: 90
FAT: 6G
CARBOHYDRATES: 4G
PROTEIN: 6G

BUFFALO CAULIFLOWER BITES

PREP TIME: 10 MINUTES | COOK TIME: 25 MINUTES
TOTAL TIME: 35 MINUTES

INGREDIENTS:

- 1 head cauliflower, cut into florets
- 1/2 cup almond flour
- 1/2 cup unsweetened almond milk
- 1 teaspoon garlic powder
- 1 teaspoon paprika
- Salt and pepper to taste
- 1/2 cup buffalo sauce
- Ranch or blue cheese dressing for dipping (optional)

INSTRUCTIONS:

1. Turn the oven on to 450°F, or 230°C. Use parchment paper to line a baking sheet.
2. To prepare a batter, combine almond flour, unsweetened almond milk, paprika, garlic powder, salt, and pepper in a basin.
3. After uniformly coating each cauliflower floret with batter, transfer it to the baking sheet that has been prepared.
4. Bake the cauliflower for 20 to 25 minutes or until it's crispy and golden brown.
5. After taking the cauliflower out of the oven, slather it evenly with buffalo sauce.
6. Place the cauliflower back on the baking pan and continue baking for five more minutes.
7. If preferred, serve hot with ranch or blue cheese dressing for dipping.

NUTRITIONAL INFORMATION:

(PER SERVING, ABOUT 4 SERVINGS TOTAL)
CALORIES: 120
FAT: 6G
CARBOHYDRATES: 10G
PROTEIN: 5G

MINI BELL PEPPER NACHOS

PREP TIME: 15 MINUTES | COOK TIME: 10 MINUTES
TOTAL TIME: 25 MINUTES

INGREDIENTS:

- 6 mini bell peppers, halved and seeds removed
- 1/2 cup shredded cheddar cheese
- 1/4 cup diced tomatoes
- 1/4 cup sliced black olives
- 1/4 cup diced red onion
- 1/4 cup chopped fresh cilantro
- Guacamole, sour cream, and salsa for serving (optional)

INSTRUCTIONS:

1. Set oven temperature to 400°F or 200°C. Use parchment paper to line a baking sheet.

2. Place the small bell pepper halves, cut side up, on the baking sheet that has been prepared.
3. Chopped tomatoes, sliced black olives, chopped red onion, and shredded cheddar cheese should be stuffed into each pepper half.
4. Bake the cheese for 8 to 10 minutes or until it bubbles and melts.
5. Take out of the oven and top with freshly cut cilantro.
6. If preferred, serve immediately with salsa, sour cream, and guacamole.

NUTRITIONAL INFORMATION:
(PER SERVING, ABOUT 4 SERVINGS TOTAL)
CALORIES: 90
FAT: 6G
CARBOHYDRATES: 6G
PROTEIN: 4G

SPINACH AND ARTICHOKE DIP STUFFED MUSHROOMS
PREP TIME: 15 MINUTES | COOK TIME: 20 MINUTES
TOTAL TIME: 35 MINUTES

INGREDIENTS:
- 12 large mushrooms, stems removed
- 1 cup spinach, chopped
- 1/2 cup artichoke hearts, chopped
- 1/4 cup grated Parmesan cheese
- 1/4 cup cream cheese, softened
- 1/4 cup shredded mozzarella cheese
- 1 clove garlic, minced
- Salt and pepper to taste

INSTRUCTIONS:
1. Turn the oven on to 375°F, or 190°C. Use parchment paper to line a baking sheet.
2. When the baking sheet is ready, place the mushroom caps cavity-side up.
3. Combine chopped artichoke hearts, chopped spinach, melted cream cheese, grated Parmesan cheese, shredded mozzarella cheese, minced garlic, salt, and pepper in a bowl.
4. Pour a liberal amount of the spinach and artichoke dip mixture into each mushroom cap.
5. Bake for 18 to 20 minutes until the mixture is brown and bubbling and the mushrooms are soft.
6. Warm up the food.

NUTRITIONAL INFORMATION:
(PER SERVING, ABOUT 4 SERVINGS TOTAL)
CALORIES: 120
FAT: 8G
CARBOHYDRATES: 6G
PROTEIN: 7G

SMOKED SALMON CUCUMBER ROLLS

PREP TIME: 15 MINUTES | COOK TIME: 0 MINUTES
TOTAL TIME: 15 MINUTES

INGREDIENTS:

- 1 large cucumber
- 4 oz smoked salmon
- 4 oz cream cheese, softened
- 1 tablespoon fresh dill, chopped
- 1 tablespoon capers (optional)
- Lemon wedges for serving (optional)

INSTRUCTIONS:

1. A mandoline slicer or vegetable peeler may cut the cucumber into thin, lengthwise slices.
2. Combine chopped fresh dill and softened cream cheese in a small bowl.
3. Apply a thin coating of the cream cheese mixture on each cucumber strip.
4. Put a smoked salmon slice over the cream cheese.
5. Top with capers, if desired.
6. Roll the cucumber strips with the cream cheese and salmon mixture.
7. If needed, use a toothpick to secure each roll.
8. If preferred, serve right away with lemon slices.

NUTRITIONAL INFORMATION:

(PER SERVING, ABOUT 4 SERVINGS TOTAL)
CALORIES: 110
FAT: 8G
CARBOHYDRATES: 3G
PROTEIN: 7G

DEVILED EGGS WITH AVOCADO

PREP TIME: 15 MINUTES | COOK TIME: 10 MINUTES
TOTAL TIME: 25 MINUTES

INGREDIENTS:

- 6 hard-boiled eggs, peeled and halved
- 1 ripe avocado
- 2 tablespoons mayonnaise
- 1 teaspoon Dijon mustard
- 1 teaspoon lemon juice
- Salt and pepper to taste
- Paprika and chopped chives for garnish

INSTRUCTIONS:

1. Hard-boiled eggs should be cut in half, and the yolks should be removed and put in a basin.
2. Mashing ripe avocado, mayonnaise, Dijon mustard, lemon juice, salt, and pepper achieves smooth and creamy yolks.
3. Re-spoon the avocado mixture into each half of the egg white.

4. As a garnish, add chopped chives and paprika.
5. Serve right away or put in the fridge until you're ready to serve.

NUTRITIONAL INFORMATION:
(PER SERVING, ABOUT 4 SERVINGS TOTAL)
CALORIES: 140
FAT: 12G
CARBOHYDRATES: 3G
PROTEIN: 6G

GREEK YOGURT RANCH VEGGIE DIP CUPS

PREP TIME: 10 MINUTES | COOK TIME: 0 MINUTES
TOTAL TIME: 10 MINUTES

INGREDIENTS:
- 1 cup Greek yogurt
- 1 tablespoon ranch seasoning mix
- Assorted raw vegetables (carrots, celery, bell peppers, cucumbers, etc.) for dipping

INSTRUCTIONS:
1. Blend the ranch seasoning mix and Greek yoghurt in a bowl until well blended.
2. Divide the ranch dip into ramekins or little cups.
3. Place a variety of raw veggies in a circle around the dip cups.
4. Serve right away.

NUTRITIONAL INFORMATION:
(PER SERVING, ABOUT 4 SERVINGS TOTAL)
CALORIES: 60
FAT: 2G
CARBOHYDRATES: 4G
PROTEIN: 8G

SPICY CHICKEN LETTUCE WRAPS

PREP TIME: 15 MINUTES | COOK TIME: 15 MINUTES
TOTAL TIME: 30 MINUTES

INGREDIENTS:
- 1 lb ground chicken
- 1 tablespoon olive oil
- 1/2 onion, diced
- 2 cloves garlic, minced
- 1 bell pepper, diced
- 1 tablespoon soy sauce
- 1 tablespoon sriracha sauce
- 1 teaspoon ground ginger
- Salt and pepper to taste

- Iceberg or butter lettuce leaves for wrapping
- Sliced green onions and sesame seeds for garnish

INSTRUCTIONS:

1. In a big skillet over medium heat, warm up the olive oil.
2. Simmer the chopped onion and minced garlic in the pan until they are tender.
3. Using a spoon, break up the ground chicken as it cooks until it is browned and well-cooked. Add the chicken to the skillet.
4. Add the ground ginger, soy sauce, sriracha sauce, sliced bell pepper, salt, and pepper. Simmer for two to three minutes more.
5. Spoon the hot chicken mixture onto the leaves of the lettuce.
6. Add sesame seeds and sliced green onions as garnish.
7. Serve right away.

NUTRITIONAL INFORMATION:

(PER SERVING, ABOUT 4 SERVINGS TOTAL)
CALORIES: 220
FAT: 12G
CARBOHYDRATES: 5G
PROTEIN: 22G

GRILLED CHICKEN CAESAR SALAD

PREP TIME: 15 MINUTES | COOK TIME: 15 MINUTES
TOTAL TIME: 30 MINUTES

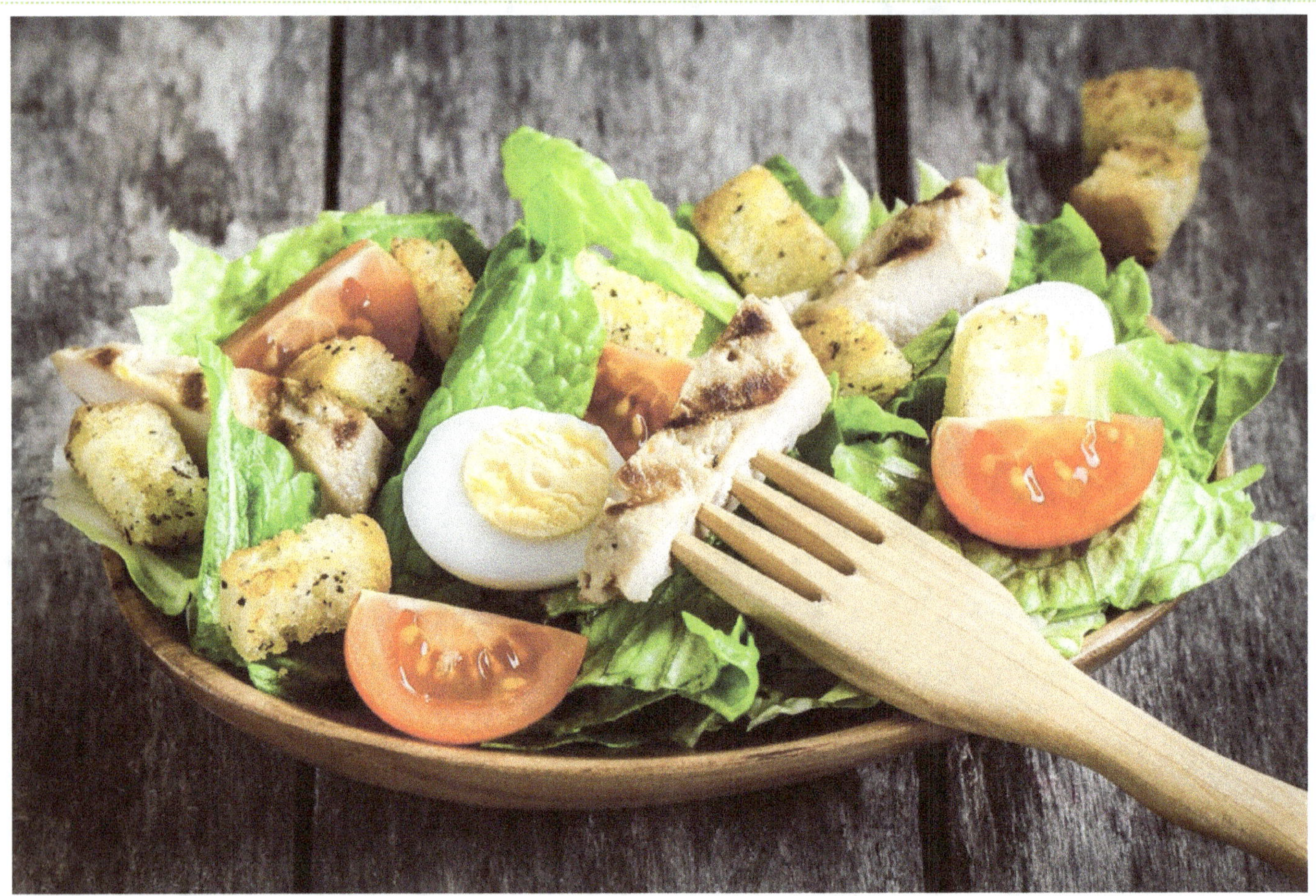

INGREDIENTS:
- 2 boneless, skinless chicken breasts
- Salt and pepper to taste
- 1 tablespoon olive oil
- 1 head romaine lettuce, chopped
- 1/2 cup Caesar dressing
- 1/4 cup grated Parmesan cheese
- Croutons for serving (optional)

INSTRUCTIONS:
1. Turn the heat up to medium-high on a grill or grill pan.
2. Add olive oil, salt, and pepper to the chicken breasts.
3. The chicken breasts should be cooked through and no longer pink in the middle after grilling them for 6–7 minutes on each side.
4. After a few minutes of rest, finely slice the chicken.
5. Toss chopped romaine lettuce with Caesar dressing in a large basin until well covered.

6. Arrange the prepared lettuce on individual serving dishes.
7. Place sliced grilled chicken on top of each platter.
8. Top with grated Parmesan cheese.
9. If preferred, top with croutons and serve right away.

NUTRITIONAL INFORMATION:
(PER SERVING, ABOUT 4 SERVINGS TOTAL)
CALORIES: 300
FAT: 20G
CARBOHYDRATES: 4G
PROTEIN: 25G

AVOCADO AND BACON SPINACH SALAD
PREP TIME: 10 MINUTES | COOK TIME: 10 MINUTES
TOTAL TIME: 20 MINUTES

INGREDIENTS:
- 6 cups baby spinach leaves
- 4 slices bacon, cooked and crumbled
- 2 ripe avocados, diced
- 1/4 cup sliced red onion
- 1/4 cup chopped walnuts
- 2 tablespoons balsamic vinegar
- 2 tablespoons olive oil
- Salt and pepper to taste

INSTRUCTIONS:
1. Combine baby spinach leaves, crumbled bacon, diced avocados, sliced red onion, and chopped walnuts in a big bowl.
2. To create the dressing, combine the olive oil, salt, pepper, and balsamic vinegar in a small bowl.
3. After drizzling the salad with the dressing, gently toss to coat.
4. Serve right away.

NUTRITIONAL INFORMATION:
(PER SERVING, ABOUT 4 SERVINGS TOTAL)
CALORIES: 280
FAT: 24G
CARBOHYDRATES: 11G
PROTEIN: 7G

GREEK SALAD WITH FETA AND OLIVES

PREP TIME: 15 MINUTES | COOK TIME: 0 MINUTES
TOTAL TIME: 15 MINUTES

INGREDIENTS:

- 4 cups chopped Romaine lettuce
- 1 cucumber, diced
- 1 cup cherry tomatoes, halved
- 1/2 cup sliced red onion
- 1/2 cup Kalamata olives
- 1/2 cup crumbled feta cheese
- 1/4 cup extra virgin olive oil
- 2 tablespoons red wine vinegar
- 1 teaspoon dried oregano
- Salt and pepper to taste

INSTRUCTIONS:

1. Chopped Romaine lettuce, diced cucumber, split cherry tomatoes, sliced red onion, Kalamata olives, and crumbled feta cheese should all be combined in a big bowl.
2. To create the dressing, combine the dried oregano, extra virgin olive oil, red wine vinegar, salt, and pepper in a small dish.
3. After drizzling the salad with the dressing, gently toss to coat.
4. Serve right away.

NUTRITIONAL INFORMATION:

(PER SERVING, ABOUT 4 SERVINGS TOTAL)
CALORIES: 240
FAT: 20G
CARBOHYDRATES: 9G
PROTEIN: 6G

SHRIMP AND AVOCADO COBB SALAD

PREP TIME: 20 MINUTES | COOK TIME: 5 MINUTES
TOTAL TIME: 25 MINUTES

INGREDIENTS:

- 1 lb large shrimp, peeled and deveined
- Salt and pepper to taste
- 2 tablespoons olive oil
- 6 cups mixed salad greens
- 2 ripe avocados, diced
- 1 cup cherry tomatoes, halved
- 4 slices bacon, cooked and crumbled
- 2 hard-boiled eggs, sliced
- 1/2 cup crumbled blue cheese
- 1/4 cup ranch dressing

INSTRUCTIONS:

1. Add a little salt and pepper to the shrimp.
2. In a pan over medium heat, warm the olive oil.
3. When the shrimp are pink and fully cooked, add them to the skillet and cook for two to three minutes on each side.
4. Mix salad greens in a big basin.
5. On top of the mixed greens, add diced avocado, halved cherry tomatoes, cooked and crumbled bacon, hard-boiled egg slices, crumbled blue cheese, and cooked shrimp.
6. Over the salad, drizzle some ranch dressing.
7. Serve right away.

NUTRITIONAL INFORMATION:

(PER SERVING, ABOUT 4 SERVINGS TOTAL)
CALORIES: 380
FAT: 28G
CARBOHYDRATES: 12G
PROTEIN: 22G

BROCCOLI CAULIFLOWER SALAD WITH LEMON DRESSING

PREP TIME: 15 MINUTES | COOK TIME: 0 MINUTES
TOTAL TIME: 15 MINUTES

INGREDIENTS:

- 2 cups broccoli florets
- 2 cups cauliflower florets
- 1/4 cup diced red onion
- 1/4 cup chopped fresh parsley
- 1/4 cup chopped walnuts
- 1/4 cup raisins or dried cranberries
- 1/4 cup mayonnaise
- 2 tablespoons lemon juice
- 1 tablespoon Dijon mustard
- Salt and pepper to taste

INSTRUCTIONS:

1. Combine broccoli and cauliflower florets, diced red onion, chopped walnuts, chopped fresh parsley, and raisins or dried cranberries in a big bowl.
2. Combine the mayonnaise, lemon juice, Dijon mustard, salt, and pepper in a small bowl to create the dressing.
3. Drizzle the salad with the dressing and gently mix to coat.
4. Serve right away.

NUTRITIONAL INFORMATION:

(PER SERVING, ABOUT 4 SERVINGS TOTAL)
CALORIES: 220
FAT: 18G

CARBOHYDRATES: 14G
PROTEIN: 4G

THAI BEEF SALAD WITH PEANUT DRESSING

PREP TIME: 15 MINUTES | COOK TIME: 10 MINUTES
TOTAL TIME: 25 MINUTES

INGREDIENTS:

- 1 lb flank steak
- Salt and pepper to taste
- 6 cups mixed salad greens
- 1 cucumber, thinly sliced
- 1 bell pepper, thinly sliced
- 1/4 cup chopped peanuts
- Fresh cilantro leaves for garnish

PEANUT DRESSING:

- 1/4 cup creamy peanut butter
- 2 tablespoons soy sauce
- 2 tablespoons lime juice
- 1 tablespoon sesame oil
- 1 tablespoon honey
- 1 teaspoon grated ginger
- 1 clove garlic, minced
- Water to thin, if needed

INSTRUCTIONS:

1. Add salt and pepper to the flank steak to season it.
2. Grill pans or grills are heated to medium-high heat. Cook the steak until it reaches the desired level of doneness, 4–5 minutes on each side. After a few minutes of resting, thinly slice against the grain.
3. Combine bell pepper, cucumber, and mixed salad greens in a big bowl.
4. Combine all the peanut dressing ingredients in another bowl and whisk until well combined. If necessary, thin the dressing with water.
5. Place the cut meat over the greens.
6. Over the salad and meat, pour the peanut dressing.
7. Add chopped peanuts and fresh cilantro leaves as garnish.
8. Serve right away.

NUTRITIONAL INFORMATION:

(PER SERVING, ABOUT 4 SERVINGS TOTAL)
CALORIES: 350
FAT: 21G
CARBOHYDRATES: 15G
PROTEIN: 28G

CAPRESE SALAD WITH BALSAMIC GLAZE

PREP TIME: 10 MINUTES | COOK TIME: 0 MINUTES
TOTAL TIME: 10 MINUTES

INGREDIENTS:

- 2 large tomatoes, sliced
- 8 oz fresh mozzarella cheese, sliced
- Fresh basil leaves
- Balsamic glaze
- Salt and pepper to taste

INSTRUCTIONS:

1. On a serving dish, arrange tomato and mozzarella cheese slices in succession.
2. Place a few fresh basil leaves in between the mozzarella and tomato slices.
3. Over the salad, drizzle some balsamic glaze.
4. To taste, add salt and pepper for seasoning.
5. Serve right away.

NUTRITIONAL INFORMATION:

(PER SERVING, ABOUT 4 SERVINGS TOTAL)
CALORIES: 200
FAT: 14G
CARBOHYDRATES: 8G
PROTEIN: 12G

TACO SALAD WITH GROUND TURKEY

PREP TIME: 15 MINUTES | COOK TIME: 15 MINUTES
TOTAL TIME: 30 MINUTES

INGREDIENTS:

- 1 lb ground turkey
- 1 tablespoon olive oil
- 1 packet of taco seasoning
- 6 cups chopped romaine lettuce
- 1 cup cherry tomatoes, halved
- 1 cup shredded cheddar cheese
- 1 avocado, diced
- 1/2 cup salsa
- 1/4 cup sour cream
- Tortilla chips for serving (optional)

INSTRUCTIONS:

1. Warm the olive oil in a pan over medium heat. Break up the ground turkey with a spoon while you cook it until it becomes brown.
2. Add taco seasoning and heat as directed on the box.
3. Diced avocado, cooked ground turkey, cherry tomatoes, shredded cheddar cheese, and romaine lettuce should all be combined in a big dish.

4. Add sour cream and salsa to the salad and toss.
5. If preferred, top with tortilla chips and serve right away.

NUTRITIONAL INFORMATION:
(PER SERVING, ABOUT 4 SERVINGS TOTAL)
CALORIES: 400
FAT: 25G
CARBOHYDRATES: 15G
PROTEIN: 30G

CREAMY CAULIFLOWER SOUP WITH CRISPY BACON
PREP TIME: 10 MINUTES | COOK TIME: 25 MINUTES
TOTAL TIME: 35 MINUTES

INGREDIENTS:
- 1 head cauliflower, chopped into florets
- 1 onion, chopped
- 2 cloves garlic, minced
- 4 cups chicken or vegetable broth
- 1/2 cup heavy cream
- Salt and pepper to taste
- 4 slices bacon, cooked and crumbled
- Chopped chives for garnish

INSTRUCTIONS:
1. Diced onion and minced garlic should be cooked in a big saucepan until tender.
2. Toss the chopped cauliflower florets and pour in the chicken or vegetable broth. After boiling it, decrease the heat and simmer the cauliflower for approximately 20 minutes or until it is soft.
3. Blend the soup with an immersion blender until it's smooth. Alternately, pour the soup back into the pot after transferring it in stages to a blender and blending until smooth.
4. Add heavy cream and season to taste with salt and pepper.
5. Garnish the heated soup with chopped chives and crumbled bacon.

NUTRITIONAL INFORMATION:
(PER SERVING, ABOUT 4 SERVINGS TOTAL)
CALORIES: 220
FAT: 15G
CARBOHYDRATES: 12G
PROTEIN: 8G

CHICKEN ZOODLE SOUP

PREP TIME: 10 MINUTES | COOK TIME: 25 MINUTES
TOTAL TIME: 35 MINUTES

INGREDIENTS:

- 1 tablespoon olive oil
- 1 onion, diced
- 2 carrots, diced
- 2 celery stalks, diced
- 2 cloves garlic, minced
- 6 cups chicken broth
- 2 cups cooked shredded chicken
- 2 medium zucchinis, spiralized into noodles
- Salt and pepper to taste
- Chopped parsley for garnish

INSTRUCTIONS:

1. In a large saucepan, heat the olive oil over medium heat. Add the minced garlic, chopped onion, carrots, and celery. Sauté the food until it becomes tender.
2. After adding the chicken broth, boil the mixture.
3. Simmer the cooked, shredded chicken in the saucepan for ten minutes.
4. When the zucchini noodles are ready, add them to the stew and simmer for five minutes.
5. To taste, add salt and pepper for seasoning.
6. Garnish the heated soup with minced parsley.

NUTRITIONAL INFORMATION:

(PER SERVING, ABOUT 4 SERVINGS TOTAL)
CALORIES: 200
FAT: 8G
CARBOHYDRATES: 8G
PROTEIN: 20G

TOMATO BASIL SOUP WITH PARMESAN CRISPS

PREP TIME: 10 MINUTES | COOK TIME: 30 MINUTES
TOTAL TIME: 40 MINUTES

INGREDIENTS:

- 2 tablespoons olive oil
- 1 onion, chopped
- 2 cloves garlic, minced
- 28 oz canned whole tomatoes
- 2 cups vegetable broth
- 1/2 cup fresh basil leaves
- Salt and pepper to taste
- 1/2 cup grated Parmesan cheese

INSTRUCTIONS:

1. In a big saucepan, warm the olive oil over medium heat. Add the onion and garlic when they are minced and softened and sauté.
2. Add vegetable broth and canned whole tomatoes with their juices to the saucepan. Simmer and cook for around 20 minutes.
3. Puree the soup with an immersion blender until it's smooth. Alternately, pour the soup back into the pot after transferring it in stages to a blender and blending until smooth.
4. Add the fresh basil leaves and season to taste with salt and pepper.
5. Set the oven to 400°F or 200°C. Line a baking sheet with parchment paper. Place grate Parmesan cheese spoonfuls onto the baking sheet and gently flatten them. Bake until crispy and golden, 5 to 7 minutes.
6. Serve the hot tomato basil soup with Parmesan chips on top.

NUTRITIONAL INFORMATION:
(PER SERVING, ABOUT 4 SERVINGS TOTAL)
CALORIES: 180
FAT: 10G
CARBOHYDRATES: 15G
PROTEIN: 8G

SPINACH AND SAUSAGE SOUP
PREP TIME: 10 MINUTES | COOK TIME: 25 MINUTES
TOTAL TIME: 35 MINUTES

INGREDIENTS:
- 1 tablespoon olive oil
- 1 lb Italian sausage, casings removed
- 1 onion, chopped
- 2 cloves garlic, minced
- 4 cups chicken broth
- 1 can (14 oz) diced tomatoes
- 4 cups fresh spinach leaves
- Salt and pepper to taste
- Grated Parmesan cheese for garnish

INSTRUCTIONS:
1. In a big saucepan, warm up the olive oil over medium heat. Break up the Italian sausage with a spoon while it cooks until it becomes brown.
2. Add minced garlic and diced onion to the saucepan. Once the onion is transparent, sauté it.
3. Add the diced tomatoes with their juices and the chicken broth. Simmer for around fifteen minutes.
4. Cook until the fresh spinach leaves wilt by stirring them in.
5. To taste, add salt and pepper for seasoning.
6. Serve the hot sausage and spinach soup with grated Parmesan cheese on top.

NUTRITIONAL INFORMATION:
(PER SERVING, ABOUT 4 SERVINGS TOTAL)
CALORIES: 320
FAT: 20G
CARBOHYDRATES: 10G

KETO BROCCOLI CHEESE SOUP

PREP TIME: 10 MINUTES | COOK TIME: 25 MINUTES
TOTAL TIME: 35 MINUTES

INGREDIENTS:

- 2 tablespoons butter
- 1 onion, chopped
- 2 cloves garlic, minced
- 4 cups chopped broccoli florets
- 4 cups chicken broth
- 1 cup heavy cream
- 2 cups shredded cheddar cheese
- Salt and pepper to taste
- Crispy bacon for garnish (optional)

INSTRUCTIONS:

1. Melt butter in a large saucepan over medium heat. Add the onion and garlic when they are minced and softened and sauté.
2. Toss in the chopped broccoli florets. After adding the chicken broth, boil the mixture. Simmer broccoli for 15 minutes or until it is soft.
3. Blend the soup with an immersion blender until it's smooth. Alternately, pour the soup back into the pot after transferring it in stages to a blender and blending until smooth.
4. Stir in the heavy cream and cheddar shreds once the cheese has melted and the soup has become creamy.
5. To taste, add salt and pepper for seasoning.
6. If preferred, top the hot keto broccoli cheese soup with crispy bacon.

NUTRITIONAL INFORMATION:

(PER SERVING, ABOUT 4 SERVINGS TOTAL)
CALORIES: 450
FAT: 36G
CARBOHYDRATES: 10G
PROTEIN: 20G

SPICY THAI COCONUT CHICKEN SOUP

PREP TIME: 10 MINUTES | COOK TIME: 20 MINUTES
TOTAL TIME: 30 MINUTES

INGREDIENTS:

- 1 tablespoon coconut oil
- 1 lb boneless, skinless chicken breasts, thinly sliced
- 1 onion, sliced
- 2 cloves garlic, minced
- 1 red bell pepper, sliced

- 1 can (14 oz) coconut milk
- 4 cups chicken broth
- 2 tablespoons Thai red curry paste
- 1 tablespoon fish sauce
- 1 tablespoon lime juice
- 2 tablespoons chopped cilantro for garnish
- Sliced red chilli for garnish (optional)

INSTRUCTIONS:

1. Warm the coconut oil in a large saucepan set over medium heat. When the chicken breasts are browned, add them sliced.
2. Add the minced garlic, onion, and red bell pepper slices to the saucepan. Sauté the veggies until they are tender.
3. Add the chicken broth and coconut milk. Stir in lime juice, fish sauce, and Thai red curry paste. Simmer and cook for around ten minutes.
4. Top the hot, spicy Thai coconut chicken soup with sliced red chile and chopped cilantro.

NUTRITIONAL INFORMATION:

(PER SERVING, ABOUT 4 SERVINGS TOTAL)
CALORIES: 320
FAT: 20G
CARBOHYDRATES: 8G
PROTEIN: 25G

MEXICAN CHICKEN AVOCADO LIME SOUP

PREP TIME: 10 MINUTES | COOK TIME: 25 MINUTES
TOTAL TIME: 35 MINUTES

INGREDIENTS:

- 1 tablespoon olive oil
- 1 onion, chopped
- 2 cloves garlic, minced
- 1 lb boneless, skinless chicken breasts, diced
- 1 can (14 oz) diced tomatoes
- 4 cups chicken broth
- 1 teaspoon ground cumin
- 1 teaspoon chilli powder
- 2 tablespoons lime juice
- 1 avocado, diced
- Chopped cilantro for garnish
- Sliced jalapeño for garnish (optional)

INSTRUCTIONS:

1. In a big saucepan, warm the olive oil over medium heat. Add the onion and garlic when they are minced and softened and sauté.
2. To the saucepan, add the chopped chicken breasts. Cook until every side is browned.
3. Add the ground cumin, chilli powder, chopped tomatoes, and chicken broth. Simmer for around fifteen minutes.

4. Add the cubed avocado and lime juice just before serving.
5. Garnish the spicy Mexican chicken avocado lime soup with sliced jalapeño and chopped cilantro, if preferred.

NUTRITIONAL INFORMATION:
(PER SERVING, ABOUT 4 SERVINGS TOTAL)
CALORIES: 280
FAT: 14G
CARBOHYDRATES: 10G
PROTEIN: 25G

CREAMY MUSHROOM SOUP WITH GARLIC AND THYME

PREP TIME: 10 MINUTES | COOK TIME: 25 MINUTES
TOTAL TIME: 35 MINUTES

INGREDIENTS:
- 2 tablespoons butter
- 1 onion, chopped
- 2 cloves garlic, minced
- 1 lb mushrooms, sliced
- 4 cups vegetable broth
- 1 cup heavy cream
- 2 teaspoons fresh thyme leaves
- Salt and pepper to taste
- Chopped parsley for garnish

INSTRUCTIONS:
1. Melt butter in a large saucepan over medium heat. Add the onion and garlic when they are minced and softened and sauté.
2. To the saucepan, add the sliced mushrooms. Simmer them until the liquid evaporates, and they soften.
3. After adding the vegetable broth, boil the mixture. Simmer for around fifteen minutes.
4. Add the fresh thyme leaves and heavy cream and stir. To taste, add salt and pepper for seasoning.
5. Garnish the hot, creamy mushroom soup with chopped parsley.

NUTRITIONAL INFORMATION:
(PER SERVING, ABOUT 4 SERVINGS TOTAL)
CALORIES: 280
FAT: 24G
CARBOHYDRATES: 10G
PROTEIN: 6G

GARLIC BUTTER ROASTED BRUSSELS SPROUTS

PREP TIME: 10 MINUTES | COOK TIME: 25 MINUTES
TOTAL TIME: 35 MINUTES

INGREDIENTS:

- 1 lb Brussels sprouts, trimmed and halved
- 2 tablespoons olive oil
- 2 cloves garlic, minced
- Salt and pepper to taste
- 2 tablespoons unsalted butter, melted

INSTRUCTIONS:

1. Set oven temperature to 400°F or 200°C.
2. After being tossed in a big basin with olive oil, minced garlic, salt, and pepper, Brussels sprouts should be equally covered.
3. Arrange the Brussels sprouts on a baking sheet in a single layer.
4. Roast the Brussels sprouts in a preheated oven for 20 to 25 minutes, tossing halfway through or until they are soft and golden.
5. Before serving, drizzle the roasted Brussels sprouts with melted butter.

NUTRITIONAL INFORMATION:

(PER SERVING, ABOUT 4 SERVINGS TOTAL)
CALORIES: 120
FAT: 10G
CARBOHYDRATES: 7G
PROTEIN: 3G

PARMESAN ROASTED ASPARAGUS SPEARS

PREP TIME: 5 MINUTES | COOK TIME: 15 MINUTES
TOTAL TIME: 20 MINUTES

INGREDIENTS:

- 1 lb asparagus spears, trimmed
- 2 tablespoons olive oil
- Salt and pepper to taste
- 1/4 cup grated Parmesan cheese

INSTRUCTIONS:

1. Set the oven temperature to 425°F (220°C).
2. Arrange the asparagus spears on a baking sheet. Drizzle with olive oil and season with pepper and salt. Toss for an even coat.
3. On top of the asparagus, scatter the grated Parmesan cheese.

4. Roast for 12 to 15 minutes in a preheated oven or until the asparagus is soft and the Parmesan is crispy and golden.

NUTRITIONAL INFORMATION:
(PER SERVING, ABOUT 4 SERVINGS TOTAL)
CALORIES: 90
FAT: 7G
CARBOHYDRATES: 4G
PROTEIN: 4G

CAULIFLOWER MASH WITH CHIVES

PREP TIME: 10 MINUTES | COOK TIME: 15 MINUTES
TOTAL TIME: 25 MINUTES

INGREDIENTS:
- 1 head cauliflower, cut into florets
- 2 cloves garlic, minced
- 2 tablespoons unsalted butter
- Salt and pepper to taste
- 2 tablespoons chopped fresh chives

INSTRUCTIONS:
1. Heat a large saucepan of salted water until it boils. Add minced garlic and cauliflower florets to the saucepan. Cook the cauliflower for ten to twelve minutes, or until it is very soft.
2. After draining, place the cauliflower in a blender or food processor.
3. Season the cauliflower with salt, pepper, and unsalted butter. Blend till creamy and smooth.
4. Add chopped fresh chives and stir.
5. Hot cauliflower mash should be served.

NUTRITIONAL INFORMATION:
(PER SERVING, ABOUT 4 SERVINGS TOTAL)
CALORIES: 70
FAT: 5G
CARBOHYDRATES: 6G
PROTEIN: 3G

LEMON GARLIC GREEN BEANS

PREP TIME: 5 MINUTES | COOK TIME: 10 MINUTES
TOTAL TIME: 15 MINUTES

INGREDIENTS:

- 1 lb green beans, trimmed
- 2 tablespoons olive oil
- 2 cloves garlic, minced
- Zest of 1 lemon
- Salt and pepper to taste
- Lemon wedges for serving (optional)

INSTRUCTIONS:

1. In a big skillet over medium heat, warm up the olive oil. When aromatic, add the minced garlic and simmer.
2. Heat the skillet with the green beans. Sauté the green beans for 8 to 10 minutes, stirring often, or until soft but still crunchy.
3. Mix in the zest from the lemon and add salt and pepper according to taste.
4. Warm up the lemon-garlic green beans and, if preferred, serve them with slices of lemon.

NUTRITIONAL INFORMATION:

(PER SERVING, ABOUT 4 SERVINGS TOTAL)
CALORIES: 80
FAT: 5G
CARBOHYDRATES: 8G
PROTEIN: 2G

CHEESY BAKED ZUCCHINI STICKS

PREP TIME: 10 MINUTES | COOK TIME: 20 MINUTES
TOTAL TIME: 30 MINUTES

INGREDIENTS:

- 2 large zucchini, cut into sticks
- 1/2 cup grated Parmesan cheese
- 1/2 cup panko breadcrumbs
- 1 teaspoon Italian seasoning
- Salt and pepper to taste
- 1 egg, beaten
- Marinara sauce for dipping (optional)

INSTRUCTIONS:

1. Set the oven temperature to 425°F (220°C). Use parchment paper to line a baking sheet.
2. Grated Parmesan cheese, panko breadcrumbs, Italian seasoning, salt, and pepper should all be combined in a shallow dish.
3. Coat the zucchini sticks in the breadcrumb mixture after dipping them into the beaten egg.
4. Arrange the coated zucchini sticks in a single layer on the baking sheet that has been ready.
5. Bake in a preheated oven for 18 to 20 minutes, or until golden and crispy.

6. Warm up the cheesy baked zucchini sticks and, if preferred, serve with marinara sauce for dipping.

NUTRITIONAL INFORMATION:
(PER SERVING, ABOUT 4 SERVINGS TOTAL)
CALORIES: 120
FAT: 5G
CARBOHYDRATES: 12G
PROTEIN: 7G

CREAMY SPINACH AND MUSHROOM GRATIN
PREP TIME: 15 MINUTES | COOK TIME: 25 MINUTES
TOTAL TIME: 40 MINUTES

INGREDIENTS:
- 1 lb fresh spinach, washed and trimmed
- 8 oz mushrooms, sliced
- 2 tablespoons butter
- 2 cloves garlic, minced
- 1 cup heavy cream
- 1/2 cup grated Parmesan cheese
- Salt and pepper to taste
- 1/4 cup breadcrumbs (optional)

INSTRUCTIONS:
1. Turn the oven on to 375°F, or 190°C. Coat a baking dish with oil.
2. Melt butter in a large skillet over medium heat. Add the chopped garlic and the sliced mushrooms, and cook until the mushrooms are soft.
3. Fill the pan with new spinach. Cook until wilted, about 3 minutes.
4. Add grated Parmesan cheese and heavy cream, and stir. Simmer until the sauce begins to thicken slightly. To taste, add salt and pepper for seasoning.
5. Spoon the batter into the ready baking dish. If using, sprinkle breadcrumbs over top.
6. Bake for 20 to 25 minutes until the top is bubbly and brown in the preheated oven.
7. Warm creamy gratin with spinach and mushrooms served.

NUTRITIONAL INFORMATION:
(PER SERVING, ABOUT 4 SERVINGS TOTAL)
CALORIES: 280
FAT: 22G
CARBOHYDRATES: 10G
PROTEIN: 12G

ROASTED GARLIC CAULIFLOWER RICE

PREP TIME: 10 MINUTES | COOK TIME: 25 MINUTES
TOTAL TIME: 35 MINUTES

INGREDIENTS:

- 1 head cauliflower, cut into florets
- 2 tablespoons olive oil
- 4 cloves garlic, minced
- Salt and pepper to taste
- Chopped parsley for garnish (optional)

INSTRUCTIONS:

1. Set the oven temperature to 425°F (220°C). Use parchment paper to line a baking sheet.
2. Cauliflower florets should be placed on the ready baking sheet. Add some minced garlic and olive oil and drizzle. For an even coat, toss.
3. To taste, add salt and pepper for seasoning.
4. Roast the cauliflower in the preheated oven for 20 to 25 minutes, tossing occasionally, or until it is soft and gently browned.
5. Before serving, garnish with chopped parsley.

NUTRITIONAL INFORMATION:

(PER SERVING, ABOUT 4 SERVINGS TOTAL)
CALORIES: 90
FAT: 7G
CARBOHYDRATES: 7G
PROTEIN: 3G

BROCCOLI BACON SALAD WITH CREAMY DRESSING

PREP TIME: 15 MINUTES | COOK TIME: 10 MINUTES
TOTAL TIME: 25 MINUTES

INGREDIENTS:

- 4 cups broccoli florets
- 6 slices bacon, cooked and crumbled
- 1/4 cup red onion, finely chopped
- 1/2 cup mayonnaise
- 2 tablespoons apple cider vinegar
- 1 tablespoon granulated sugar or sweetener of choice
- Salt and pepper to taste

INSTRUCTIONS:

1. Broccoli florets, sliced red onion, and crumbled bacon should all be combined in a big bowl.
2. To prepare the dressing, combine the mayonnaise, apple cider vinegar, sugar, salt, and pepper in a small bowl.
3. After adding the dressing, toss the broccoli mixture until it is well-covered.
4. Chill for at least an hour before serving to enable the flavours to mingle.

NUTRITIONAL INFORMATION:
(PER SERVING, ABOUT 4 SERVINGS TOTAL)
CALORIES: 280
FAT: 22G
CARBOHYDRATES: 10G
PROTEIN: 12G

LEMON HERB GRILLED EGGPLANT

PREP TIME: 10 MINUTES | COOK TIME: 10 MINUTES
TOTAL TIME: 20 MINUTES

INGREDIENTS:

- 1 large eggplant, sliced into rounds
- 2 tablespoons olive oil
- 2 cloves garlic, minced
- Zest and juice of 1 lemon
- 1 teaspoon dried thyme
- Salt and pepper to taste
- Chopped fresh parsley for garnish

INSTRUCTIONS:

1. Set the grill's temperature to medium-high.
2. Mix the olive oil, dried thyme, lemon zest, lemon juice, minced garlic, salt, and pepper in a small bowl.
3. Apply the marinade of lemon and herbs on both sides of the eggplant pieces.
4. Slices of eggplant should be soft and faintly browned after grilling for 4–5 minutes on each side.
5. Place the grilled eggplant onto a plate for serving.
6. Before serving, sprinkle some freshly chopped parsley on top.

NUTRITIONAL INFORMATION:

(PER SERVING, ABOUT 4 SERVINGS TOTAL)
CALORIES: 120
FAT: 8G
CARBOHYDRATES: 12G
PROTEIN: 2G

BALSAMIC GLAZED BRUSSELS SPROUTS

PREP TIME: 10 MINUTES | COOK TIME: 25 MINUTES
TOTAL TIME: 35 MINUTES

INGREDIENTS:

- 1 lb Brussels sprouts, trimmed and halved
- 2 tablespoons olive oil
- Salt and pepper to taste
- 2 tablespoons balsamic vinegar
- 1 tablespoon honey or maple syrup
- 1/4 cup grated Parmesan cheese (optional)

INSTRUCTIONS:

1. Warm the oven to 400°F or 200°C. Place parchment paper on one side of a baking sheet.
2. Brussels sprouts should be uniformly coated with a mixture of olive oil, salt, and pepper in a big dish.
3. Arrange Brussels sprouts in a single layer on the baking sheet that has been preheated.
4. Roast, tossing occasionally, in a preheated oven for 20 to 25 minutes or until Brussels sprouts are soft and caramelized.
5. Balsamic vinegar and honey (or maple syrup) should be heated in a small saucepan over medium heat until they are reduced and thickened, which should take around five minutes.
6. After roasting the Brussels sprouts, drizzle with the balsamic glaze.
7. Before serving, if preferred, sprinkle grated Parmesan cheese on top.

NUTRITIONAL INFORMATION:

(PER SERVING, ABOUT 4 SERVINGS TOTAL)
CALORIES: 120
FAT: 7G
CARBOHYDRATES: 12G
PROTEIN: 4G

CHEESY BAKED CAULIFLOWER TOTS

PREP TIME: 20 MINUTES | COOK TIME: 25 MINUTES
TOTAL TIME: 45 MINUTES

INGREDIENTS:

- 1 head cauliflower, cut into florets
- 1/2 cup grated Parmesan cheese
- 1/2 cup shredded cheddar cheese
- 1/4 cup almond flour
- 2 eggs
- 2 cloves garlic, minced
- 1 teaspoon dried parsley
- Salt and pepper to taste
- Cooking spray

INSTRUCTIONS:

1. Set oven temperature to 400°F or 200°C. Grease a baking pan with cooking spray and line it with parchment paper.
2. Cauliflower florets should be pulsed in a food processor until they resemble rice.
3. After putting the cauliflower "rice" in a bowl that is safe to microwave for five minutes, let it cool a little.
4. Squeeze as much moisture out of the cauliflower as possible using a fresh kitchen towel or cheesecloth.
5. Combine the cauliflower, eggs, almond flour, dried parsley, minced garlic, Parmesan cheese, and salt and pepper in a large mixing basin. Blend until well blended.
6. Put the mixture on the baking sheet that has been preheated and form it into little tots.
7. Bake in a preheated oven for 20 to 25 minutes, or until golden and crispy.
8. Hot cheese-filled baked cauliflower tots should be served with your preferred dipping sauce.

NUTRITIONAL INFORMATION:
(PER SERVING, ABOUT 4 SERVINGS TOTAL)
CALORIES: 180
FAT: 11G
CARBOHYDRATES: 10G
PROTEIN: 12G

SAUTEED GARLIC BUTTER MUSHROOMS
PREP TIME: 5 MINUTES | COOK TIME: 10 MINUTES
TOTAL TIME: 15 MINUTES

INGREDIENTS:
* 1 lb mushrooms, cleaned and sliced
* 2 tablespoons butter
* 2 cloves garlic, minced
* Salt and pepper to taste
* Chopped fresh parsley for garnish (optional)

INSTRUCTIONS:
1. In a large skillet, melt butter over medium-high heat.
2. Garlic powder should be added to the pan and cooked until aromatic.
3. When the mushrooms shed their moisture and turn golden brown, add the sliced ones to the pan and simmer, turning from time to time.
4. To taste, add salt and pepper for seasoning.
5. Before serving, sprinkle some freshly chopped parsley on top.

NUTRITIONAL INFORMATION:
(PER SERVING, ABOUT 4 SERVINGS TOTAL)
CALORIES: 80
FAT: 6G
CARBOHYDRATES: 5G
PROTEIN: 3G

GREEN BEAN ALMONDINE

PREP TIME: 10 MINUTES | COOK TIME: 10 MINUTES
TOTAL TIME: 20 MINUTES

INGREDIENTS:

- 1 lb green beans, trimmed
- 2 tablespoons butter
- 1/4 cup sliced almonds
- 2 cloves garlic, minced
- 1 tablespoon lemon juice
- Salt and pepper to taste

INSTRUCTIONS:

1. Heat a big saucepan of salted water till it boils. Drain and rinse with cool water after blanching the green beans for two to three minutes.
2. Melt butter in a big skillet over a medium heat. Almond slices should be added and cooked until just toasted.
3. Garlic powder should be added to the pan and cooked until aromatic.
4. Heat the green beans in a pan and add them. Sauté the green beans for 3–4 minutes, turning often, or until they are well cooked and crisp-tender.
5. Add salt and pepper to taste and drizzle lemon juice over the green beans.
6. Hot green bean almonds should be served.

NUTRITIONAL INFORMATION:

(PER SERVING, ABOUT 4 SERVINGS TOTAL)
CALORIES: 100
FAT: 8G
CARBOHYDRATES: 6G
PROTEIN: 3G

ROSEMARY ROASTED RADISHES

PREP TIME: 10 MINUTES | COOK TIME: 25 MINUTES
TOTAL TIME: 35 MINUTES

INGREDIENTS:

- 1 lb radishes, trimmed and halved
- 2 tablespoons olive oil
- 2 teaspoons chopped fresh rosemary
- Salt and pepper to taste

INSTRUCTIONS:

1. Set oven temperature to 400°F or 200°C. Use parchment paper to line a baking sheet.
2. Toss the radishes in a large bowl with salt, pepper, olive oil, and freshly chopped rosemary until well coated.
3. Arrange the radishes on the prepared baking sheet in a single layer.
4. Roast the radishes in the oven for 20 to 25 minutes, tossing occasionally, or until soft and gently browned.

5. Warm roasted radishes with rosemary are served.

NUTRITIONAL INFORMATION:
(PER SERVING, ABOUT 4 SERVINGS TOTAL)
CALORIES: 70
FAT: 7G
CARBOHYDRATES: 3G
PROTEIN: 1G

CREAMY DIJON BRUSSELS SPROUTS
PREP TIME: 10 MINUTES | COOK TIME: 20 MINUTES
TOTAL TIME: 30 MINUTES

INGREDIENTS:
- 1 lb Brussels sprouts, trimmed and halved
- 2 tablespoons butter
- 2 cloves garlic, minced
- 1/2 cup heavy cream
- 2 tablespoons Dijon mustard
- Salt and pepper to taste
- Grated Parmesan cheese for garnish (optional)

INSTRUCTIONS:
1. Heat a big saucepan of salted water till it boils. After blanching the Brussels sprouts for three to four minutes, please remove them and wash them with cool water.
2. Melt butter in a big skillet over a medium heat. When aromatic, add the minced garlic and sauté it.
3. To the skillet, add the blanched Brussels sprouts. Cook for 5 to 7 minutes, stirring often, or until they are soft and have slightly browned edges.
4. Add Dijon mustard and heavy cream, and stir. Cook until the sauce slightly thickens, about 2 to 3 more minutes.
5. To taste, add salt and pepper for seasoning.
6. Top the hot, creamy Dijon Brussels sprouts with grated Parmesan cheese if preferred.

NUTRITIONAL INFORMATION:
(PER SERVING, ABOUT 4 SERVINGS TOTAL)
CALORIES: 180
FAT: 15G
CARBOHYDRATES: 8G
PROTEIN: 4G

LEMON PARMESAN ROASTED BROCCOLI

PREP TIME: 10 MINUTES | COOK TIME: 20 MINUTES
TOTAL TIME: 30 MINUTES

INGREDIENTS:
- 1 lb broccoli florets
- 2 tablespoons olive oil
- Zest of 1 lemon
- 2 cloves garlic, minced
- 1/4 cup grated Parmesan cheese
- Salt and pepper to taste
- Lemon wedges for serving (optional)

INSTRUCTIONS:
1. Set the oven temperature to 425°F (220°C). Use parchment paper to line a baking sheet.
2. After being tossed in a big basin with olive oil, lemon zest, chopped garlic, grated Parmesan cheese, salt, and pepper, broccoli florets should be equally coated.
3. Arrange the broccoli on the prepared baking sheet in a single layer.
4. Roast the broccoli for 15 to 20 minutes in a preheated oven or until it is soft and light brownlight brown.
5. If preferred, serve the hot broccoli roasted with lemon Parmesan and lemon wedges on the side.

NUTRITIONAL INFORMATION:
(PER SERVING, ABOUT 4 SERVINGS TOTAL)
CALORIES: 110
FAT: 8G
CARBOHYDRATES: 7G
PROTEIN: 5G

SPAGHETTI SQUASH AU GRATIN

PREP TIME: 10 MINUTES | COOK TIME: 1 HOUR
TOTAL TIME: 1 HOUR 10 MINUTES

INGREDIENTS:
- 1 spaghetti squash, halved and seeds removed
- 2 tablespoons olive oil
- Salt and pepper to taste
- 1 cup shredded cheese (such as cheddar or mozzarella)
- 1/4 cup grated Parmesan cheese
- 1/4 cup heavy cream
- 2 cloves garlic, minced
- 1 teaspoon dried thyme
- Chopped fresh parsley for garnish (optional)

INSTRUCTIONS:
1. Set oven temperature to 400°F or 200°C. Use parchment paper to line a baking sheet.
2. Season the spaghetti squash halves with salt and pepper and drizzle them with olive oil.

3. Transfer the spaghetti squash halves, cut side down, to the baking sheet that has been prepared.
4. Bake in the oven for forty to fifty minutes or until the meat is fork-tender.
5. After allowing the squash to cool, scrape the flesh into strands with a fork and place it on a baking tray.
6. In a small bowl, combine grated Parmesan cheese, heavy cream, minced garlic, dry thyme, and shredded cheese.
7. After drizzling the spaghetti squash strands with the cheese mixture, toss lightly to coat.
8. Bake for 15 to 20 minutes or until the cheese is bubbling and melted.
9. Before serving, sprinkle some freshly chopped parsley on top.

NUTRITIONAL INFORMATION:

(PER SERVING, ABOUT 4 SERVINGS TOTAL)
CALORIES: 280
FAT: 22G
CARBOHYDRATES: 14G
PROTEIN: 10G

MEDITERRANEAN CUCUMBER SALAD

PREP TIME: 15 MINUTES | COOK TIME: 0 MINUTES
TOTAL TIME: 15 MINUTES

INGREDIENTS:

- 2 large cucumbers, thinly sliced
- 1 pint cherry tomatoes, halved
- 1/4 cup red onion, thinly sliced
- 1/4 cup Kalamata olives, pitted and halved
- 1/4 cup crumbled feta cheese
- 2 tablespoons fresh lemon juice
- 2 tablespoons extra virgin olive oil
- 1 tablespoon chopped fresh parsley
- Salt and pepper to taste

INSTRUCTIONS:

1. Sliced cucumbers, half cherry tomatoes, sliced red onion, halved Kalamata olives, and crumbled feta cheese should all be combined in a big dish.
2. In a small bowl, combine the extra virgin olive oil, chopped fresh parsley, fresh lemon juice, salt, and pepper.
3. After adding the dressing, toss the cucumber salad to ensure it is uniformly coated.
4. Chill the cucumber salad with a Mediterranean flair.

NUTRITIONAL INFORMATION:

(PER SERVING, ABOUT 4 SERVINGS TOTAL)
CALORIES: 120
FAT: 9G
CARBOHYDRATES: 8G
PROTEIN: 3G

BACON-WRAPPED GREEN BEAN BUNDLES

PREP TIME: 15 MINUTES | COOK TIME: 20 MINUTES
TOTAL TIME: 35 MINUTES

INGREDIENTS:

- 1 lb green beans, trimmed
- 6 slices bacon, halved crosswise
- 2 tablespoons olive oil
- 2 tablespoons honey or maple syrup
- 1 tablespoon soy sauce
- 1 teaspoon garlic powder
- Salt and pepper to taste

INSTRUCTIONS:

1. Set oven temperature to 400°F or 200°C. Use parchment paper to line a baking sheet.
2. After dividing the green beans into equal parts, bundle them together. Place a half-slice of bacon around each bundle and fasten it with toothpicks.
3. Spread the green bean bundles with bacon on the baking sheet that has been preheated.
4. Mix the olive oil, soy sauce, honey (or maple syrup), garlic powder, salt, and pepper in a small bowl.
5. Drizzle the mixture over the bundles of green beans wrapped in bacon.
6. Bake for 15 to 20 minutes in a preheated oven or until the green beans are soft and the bacon is crispy.
7. Warm green bean bundles covered in bacon should be served.

NUTRITIONAL INFORMATION:

(PER SERVING, ABOUT 4 SERVINGS TOTAL)
CALORIES: 180
FAT: 12G
CARBOHYDRATES: 10G
PROTEIN: 8G

CREAMY GARLIC PARMESAN SPAGHETTI SQUASH

PREP TIME: 10 MINUTES | COOK TIME: 50 MINUTES
TOTAL TIME: 1 HOUR

INGREDIENTS:

- 1 spaghetti squash, halved and seeds removed
- 2 tablespoons olive oil
- Salt and pepper to taste
- 3 cloves garlic, minced
- 1 cup heavy cream
- 1/2 cup grated Parmesan cheese
- 2 tablespoons chopped fresh parsley

INSTRUCTIONS:

1. Set oven temperature to 400°F or 200°C. Use parchment paper to line a baking sheet.
2. Season the spaghetti squash halves with salt and pepper and drizzle them with olive oil.
3. Transfer the spaghetti squash halves, cut side down, to the baking sheet that has been prepared.
4. Bake in the oven for forty to fifty minutes or until the meat is fork-tender.
5. After allowing the squash to cool, scrape the flesh into strands with a fork and place it in a basin.
6. Heat the olive oil in a pan over medium heat. When aromatic, add the minced garlic and simmer.
7. Add grated Parmesan cheese and heavy cream, and stir. Simmer until the sauce begins to thicken slightly.
8. Toss to cover the spaghetti squash strands with the creamy garlic Parmesan sauce.
9. Before serving, sprinkle some freshly chopped parsley on top.

NUTRITIONAL INFORMATION:

(PER SERVING, ABOUT 4 SERVINGS TOTAL)
CALORIES: 320
FAT: 28G
CARBOHYDRATES: 12G
PROTEIN: 8G

LEMON GARLIC BUTTER SALMON

PREP TIME: 10 MINUTES | COOK TIME: 12 MINUTES
TOTAL TIME: 22 MINUTES

INGREDIENTS:

- 4 salmon fillets
- 4 tablespoons unsalted butter
- 4 cloves garlic, minced
- Zest and juice of 1 lemon
- Salt and pepper to taste
- Chopped fresh parsley for garnish (optional)

INSTRUCTIONS:

1. Turn the oven on to 375°F, or 190°C. Use parchment paper to line a baking sheet.
2. Put the salmon fillets onto the baking sheet that has been prepared.
3. Melt butter in a small pot over a medium heat. When aromatic, add the minced garlic and simmer.
4. Add the lemon juice and zest and stir. To taste, add salt and pepper for seasoning.
5. Drizzle the salmon fillets with the lemon-garlic butter mixture.
6. Bake the salmon for 10 to 12 minutes, or until it is cooked through and flake easily with a fork, in a preheated oven.
7. Before serving, sprinkle some freshly chopped parsley on top.

NUTRITIONAL INFORMATION:

(PER SERVING, ABOUT 4 SERVINGS TOTAL)
CALORIES: 300
FAT: 20G
CARBOHYDRATES: 2G
PROTEIN: 25G

KETO BEEF AND BROCCOLI STIR-FRY

PREP TIME: 15 MINUTES | COOK TIME: 15 MINUTES
TOTAL TIME: 30 MINUTES

INGREDIENTS:

- 1 lb beef sirloin, thinly sliced
- 2 tablespoons olive oil
- 4 cups broccoli florets
- 4 cloves garlic, minced
- 1/4 cup soy sauce or tamari sauce
- 2 tablespoons erythritol or sweetener of choice
- 1 tablespoon sesame oil
- 1 teaspoon grated ginger
- Sesame seeds for garnish (optional)

- Sliced green onions for garnish (optional)

INSTRUCTIONS:
1. Heat the olive oil over medium-high heat in a large skillet or wok.
2. Cook the thinly sliced meat in the pan until it becomes brown.
3. Add the grated ginger and minced garlic to the pan and heat until aromatic.
4. Add the broccoli florets and stir-fry until crisp-tender.
5. Combine the sesame oil, erythritol (or sweetener), and soy sauce in a small bowl. Over the steak and broccoli in the pan, pour the sauce.
6. Simmer for two to three minutes or until the sauce thickens, stirring regularly.
7. Before serving, garnish with sliced green onions and sesame seeds.

NUTRITIONAL INFORMATION:
(PER SERVING, ABOUT 4 SERVINGS TOTAL)
CALORIES: 280
FAT: 18G
CARBOHYDRATES: 7G
PROTEIN: 25G

CAULIFLOWER CRUST PIZZA WITH PEPPERONI
PREP TIME: 20 MINUTES | COOK TIME: 25 MINUTES
TOTAL TIME: 45 MINUTES

INGREDIENTS:
- 1 head cauliflower, riced
- 1 cup shredded mozzarella cheese
- 1/4 cup grated Parmesan cheese
- 1 egg
- 1 teaspoon Italian seasoning
- 1/2 cup pizza sauce
- 1 cup shredded mozzarella cheese (for topping)
- Pepperoni slices (or toppings of choice)

INSTRUCTIONS:
1. Set the oven temperature to 425°F (220°C). Use parchment paper to line a baking sheet.
2. Rice cauliflower in a bowl that is safe to use in the microwave for five minutes. After allowing it to cool, wrap it in a fresh kitchen towel and pat dry any remaining moisture.
3. Add the cauliflower, egg, grated Parmesan cheese, shredded mozzarella cheese, and Italian seasoning to a large mixing bowl. Blend until well blended.
4. Forming the mixture into the shape of a pizza crust, press it onto the baking sheet that has been prepared.
5. Bake for 15 minutes, or until the crust is crispy and golden, in a preheated oven.
6. After taking the dough out of the oven, cover its surface with pizza sauce.
7. After sprinkling the sauce with shredded mozzarella cheese, top with pieces of pepperoni or other preferred toppings.
8. Put the pizza back in the oven and continue baking for ten more minutes or until the cheese is bubbling and melted.
9. Pizza with cauliflower crust, sliced and served hot.

NUTRITIONAL INFORMATION:
(PER SERVING, ABOUT 4 SERVINGS TOTAL)
CALORIES: 220
FAT: 14G
CARBOHYDRATES: 9G
PROTEIN: 15G

GRILLED CHICKEN WITH AVOCADO SALSA

PREP TIME: 15 MINUTES | COOK TIME: 12 MINUTES
TOTAL TIME: 27 MINUTES

INGREDIENTS:
- 4 boneless, skinless chicken breasts
- 2 tablespoons olive oil
- Salt and pepper to taste
- 1 avocado, diced
- 1/2 cup cherry tomatoes, halved
- 1/4 cup red onion, finely chopped
- 2 tablespoons fresh cilantro, chopped
- Juice of 1 lime
- 1 tablespoon olive oil

INSTRUCTIONS:
1. Set the grill's temperature to medium-high.
2. Add salt and pepper to the chicken breasts after brushing them with olive oil.
3. The chicken should be cooked through and no longer pink in the middle after grilling it for five to six minutes on each side.
4. Place the diced avocado, chopped red onion, chopped cilantro, half of the cherry tomatoes, lime juice, and olive oil in a bowl to create the salsa.
5. Top the hot grilled chicken with avocado salsa and serve.

NUTRITIONAL INFORMATION:
(PER SERVING, ABOUT 4 SERVINGS TOTAL)
CALORIES: 320
FAT: 18G
CARBOHYDRATES: 6G
PROTEIN: 32G

ZUCCHINI NOODLES WITH PESTO AND CHERRY TOMATOES

PREP TIME: 15 MINUTES | COOK TIME: 5 MINUTES
TOTAL TIME: 20 MINUTES

INGREDIENTS:

- 4 medium zucchini, spiralized into noodles
- 1 cup cherry tomatoes, halved
- 1/4 cup prepared pesto
- 2 tablespoons olive oil
- 2 cloves garlic, minced
- Salt and pepper to taste
- Grated Parmesan cheese for garnish (optional)
- Chopped fresh basil for garnish (optional)

INSTRUCTIONS:

1. In a big skillet over medium heat, warm up the olive oil. When aromatic, add the minced garlic and simmer.
2. Toss the zucchini noodles in the oil flavoured with garlic and add them to the pan. Cook until noodles are barely soft, 2 to 3 minutes.
3. Add the halved cherry tomatoes and simmer for one to two minutes or until the tomatoes are well-cooked.
4. After taking the pan off the burner, add the prepared pesto and toss until the noodles are well-covered.
5. To taste, add salt and pepper for seasoning.
6. If preferred, top the hot zucchini noodles with chopped fresh basil and grated Parmesan cheese.

NUTRITIONAL INFORMATION:

(PER SERVING, ABOUT 4 SERVINGS TOTAL)
CALORIES: 180
FAT: 14G
CARBOHYDRATES: 10G
PROTEIN: 5G

LOW-CARB EGGPLANT LASAGNA

PREP TIME: 20 MINUTES | COOK TIME: 45 MINUTES
TOTAL TIME: 1 HOUR 5 MINUTES

INGREDIENTS:

- 2 large eggplants, sliced lengthwise
- Salt
- Olive oil
- 1 lb ground beef or Italian sausage
- 1 onion, chopped
- 3 cloves garlic, minced
- 1 (24 oz) jar of low-carb marinara sauce

- 2 cups ricotta cheese
- 1 cup shredded mozzarella cheese
- 1/4 cup grated Parmesan cheese
- Fresh basil leaves for garnish (optional)

INSTRUCTIONS:

1. Turn the oven on to 375°F, or 190°C. Butter a 9 x 13-inch baking pan.
2. Place eggplant slices on a baking sheet, sprinkle with salt, and then let for ten minutes to remove extra moisture. Using paper towels, pat dry.
3. In a pan over medium heat, warm the olive oil. Add garlic, onion, and ground beef (or Italian sausage). Cook until onions are transparent and meat is browned. Eliminate extra fat.
4. Arrange a thin layer of marinara sauce in the baking dish that has been prepared. Arrange half of the pieces of eggplant on top.
5. Arrange the eggplant slices with half the meat mixture on top, then half the ricotta cheese and the remaining marinara sauce.
6. Relayer the other ingredients, then cover everything with a layer of marinara sauce.
7. Top with grated Parmesan cheese and shredded mozzarella.
8. Bake the baking dish in a preheated oven with the foil covering it for 30 minutes. Remove the foil and continue baking for 15 more minutes until the cheese becomes golden and bubbling.
9. Before serving, let the lasagna a few minutes to rest. If desired, garnish with fresh basil leaves.

NUTRITIONAL INFORMATION:

(PER SERVING, ABOUT 6 SERVINGS TOTAL)
CALORIES: 380
FAT: 25G
CARBOHYDRATES: 15G
PROTEIN: 25G

TURKEY AND SPINACH STUFFED PORTOBELLO MUSHROOMS

PREP TIME: 15 MINUTES | COOK TIME: 20 MINUTES
TOTAL TIME: 35 MINUTES

INGREDIENTS:

- 4 large portobello mushrooms, stems removed
- 1 lb ground turkey
- 2 cups fresh spinach leaves
- 1/2 cup shredded mozzarella cheese
- 2 cloves garlic, minced
- 1/2 teaspoon dried oregano
- Salt and pepper to taste
- Olive oil for brushing

INSTRUCTIONS:

1. Turn the oven on to 375°F, or 190°C. Use parchment paper to line a baking sheet.
2. The portobello mushrooms should be placed on the preheated baking sheet, gill side up. Add salt and pepper to taste and drizzle with olive oil over the tops.

3. Brown the ground turkey in a pan over medium heat. When fragrant, add the minced garlic and dry oregano.
4. Stir in the fresh spinach leaves and cook until they wilt. Remove the pan from the heat and let it cool a bit.
5. Use a spoon to distribute the turkey and spinach mixture among the portobello mushrooms.
6. Add some shredded mozzarella cheese on top of each mushroom.
7. Bake for 15 to 20 minutes in a preheated oven or until the cheese is bubbling and melted and the mushrooms are soft.
8. Warm up the filled portobello mushrooms for serving.

NUTRITIONAL INFORMATION:

(PER SERVING, ABOUT 4 SERVINGS TOTAL)
CALORIES: 280
FAT: 15G
CARBOHYDRATES: 6G
PROTEIN: 30G

SHRIMP SCAMPI WITH ZOODLES

PREP TIME: 10 MINUTES | COOK TIME: 10 MINUTES
TOTAL TIME: 20 MINUTES

INGREDIENTS:

- 1 lb shrimp, peeled and deveined
- 4 medium zucchini, spiralized into noodles
- 4 tablespoons unsalted butter
- 4 cloves garlic, minced
- Juice of 1 lemon
- 1/4 cup dry white wine (optional)
- Salt and pepper to taste
- Chopped fresh parsley for garnish (optional)

INSTRUCTIONS:

1. In a big skillet over medium heat, melt butter. When aromatic, add the minced garlic and simmer.
2. Add the shrimp to the pan and cook for 2 to 3 minutes on each side until they are pink and opaque. Remove the shrimp from the pan and set aside.
3. Pour the lemon juice and white wine (if used) into the same skillet. Simmer and cook for one to two minutes.
4. Zoodles that have been spiralized should be added to the pan and tossed to coat with sauce. Cook until noodles are barely soft, 2 to 3 minutes.
5. Take the cooked shrimp back to the pan and mix it with the zoodles by tossing them together. To taste, add salt and pepper for seasoning.
6. Top the shrimp scampi with freshly chopped parsley and serve it hot with the zoodles if preferred.

NUTRITIONAL INFORMATION:

(PER SERVING, ABOUT 4 SERVINGS TOTAL)
CALORIES: 250
FAT: 12G
CARBOHYDRATES: 8G

KETO BUTTER CHICKEN
PREP TIME: 15 MINUTES | COOK TIME: 25 MINUTES
TOTAL TIME: 40 MINUTES

INGREDIENTS:
- 1 lb boneless, skinless chicken thighs cut into bite-sized pieces
- 2 tablespoons ghee or butter
- 1 onion, finely chopped
- 3 cloves garlic, minced
- 1 tablespoon grated ginger
- 1 tablespoon garam masala
- 1 teaspoon ground turmeric
- 1 teaspoon ground coriander
- 1/2 teaspoon ground cumin
- 1/2 teaspoon chilli powder (adjust to taste)
- 1 cup canned tomato puree
- 1/2 cup heavy cream
- Salt and pepper to taste
- Chopped fresh cilantro for garnish (optional)

INSTRUCTIONS:
1. In a large pan over medium heat, melt butter or ghee. Cook the chopped onion until it becomes tender.
2. To the skillet, add the grated ginger and minced garlic. Cook until aromatic.
3. Add the ground cumin, ground coriander, ground turmeric, ground cumin, and garam masala. Cook the spices for one to two minutes or until fragrant.
4. When the chicken pieces are cooked on both sides, add them to the pan and cook.
5. After adding the bottled tomato puree, mix it with the chicken and seasonings.
6. After lowering the heat to low, simmer the chicken for 15 to 20 minutes or until it is well-cooked and the sauce has thickened.
7. After adding the heavy cream, simmer for a further five minutes.
8. To taste, add salt and pepper for seasoning.
9. Top the hot keto butter chicken with finely chopped fresh cilantro if preferred.

NUTRITIONAL INFORMATION:
(PER SERVING, ABOUT 4 SERVINGS TOTAL)
CALORIES: 350
FAT: 24G
CARBOHYDRATES: 8G
PROTEIN: 26G

STUFFED BELL PEPPERS WITH GROUND TURKEY AND QUINOA

PREP TIME: 20 MINUTES | COOK TIME: 40 MINUTES
TOTAL TIME: 1 HOUR

INGREDIENTS:

- 4 large bell peppers, halved and seeds removed
- 1 lb ground turkey
- 1 onion, chopped
- 2 cloves garlic, minced
- 1 cup cooked quinoa
- 1 cup canned black beans, drained and rinsed
- 1 cup diced tomatoes
- 1 teaspoon ground cumin
- 1 teaspoon chilli powder
- Salt and pepper to taste
- 1 cup shredded cheddar cheese
- Chopped fresh cilantro for garnish (optional)

INSTRUCTIONS:

1. Turn the oven on to 375°F, or 190°C. Coat a baking dish with oil.
2. Cut side up and place bell pepper halves in the baking dish that has been prepped.
3. Brown the ground turkey in a pan over medium heat. Cook the minced garlic and chopped onion together until the onions become transparent.
4. Add the chopped tomatoes, black beans, cooked quinoa, chilli powder, ground cumin, and salt and pepper to taste. Cook, stirring periodically, for 5 minutes.
5. Spoon to divide the turkey and quinoa mixture between the bell pepper halves.
6. Over each filled pepper, sprinkle shredded cheddar cheese.
7. Bake the baking dish for 30 minutes in a preheated oven with the foil covering it.
8. After removing the foil, bake for a further ten minutes or until the peppers are soft and the cheese is bubbling.
9. If preferred, top the spicy-filled bell peppers with finely chopped fresh cilantro.

NUTRITIONAL INFORMATION:

(PER SERVING, ABOUT 4 SERVINGS TOTAL)
CALORIES: 380
FAT: 15G
CARBOHYDRATES: 30G
PROTEIN: 30G

SPAGHETTI SQUASH CARBONARA

PREP TIME: 15 MINUTES | COOK TIME: 50 MINUTES
TOTAL TIME: 1 HOUR 5 MINUTES

INGREDIENTS:

- 1 large spaghetti squash
- 4 slices bacon, diced
- 2 cloves garlic, minced
- 2 large eggs
- 1/2 cup grated Parmesan cheese
- Salt and pepper to taste
- Chopped fresh parsley for garnish (optional)

INSTRUCTIONS:

1. Set oven temperature to 400°F, or 200°C. Scoop out the seeds after cutting the spaghetti squash in half lengthwise.
2. Transfer the squash halves, cut side down, to a parchment paper-lined baking sheet. Bake the squash for 40 to 50 minutes in a preheated oven or until it is soft and readily punctured with a fork.
3. Cook the chopped bacon over medium heat until crispy while the squash bakes. While leaving the bacon grease in the pan, remove the bacon and put it aside.
4. When the bacon oil is in the pan, add the minced garlic and simmer until fragrant.
5. Whisk eggs and grated Parmesan cheese in a bowl.
6. After cooking the spaghetti squash, scrape the meat into strands with a fork. Add the spaghetti squash strands to the pan with the bacon oil and garlic.
7. Scatter the egg and Parmesan mixture over the pan of spaghetti squash. Cook the squash until the sauce thickens slightly, stirring briskly to coat it evenly.
8. After taking off the heat, add the cooked bacon and mix. To taste, add salt and pepper for seasoning.
9. Top the hot spaghetti squash carbonara with finely chopped fresh parsley if preferred.

NUTRITIONAL INFORMATION:

(PER SERVING, ABOUT 4 SERVINGS TOTAL)
CALORIES: 280
FAT: 18G
CARBOHYDRATES: 12G
PROTEIN: 16G

BAKED LEMON HERB CHICKEN THIGHS

PREP TIME: 10 MINUTES | COOK TIME: 30 MINUTES
TOTAL TIME: 40 MINUTES

INGREDIENTS:

- 4 bone-in, skin-on chicken thighs
- 2 tablespoons olive oil
- Zest and juice of 1 lemon
- 2 cloves garlic, minced
- 1 teaspoon dried thyme
- 1 teaspoon dried rosemary
- Salt and pepper to taste
- Chopped fresh parsley for garnish (optional)

INSTRUCTIONS:

1. Set oven temperature to 400°F, or 200°C. Use parchment paper to line a baking sheet.
2. Using paper towels, pat the chicken thighs dry before arranging them on the baking sheet that has been ready.
3. Mix the olive oil, lemon zest, lemon juice, minced garlic, dried thyme, and dried rosemary in a small bowl.
4. Toss to coat the chicken thighs evenly with the lemon-herb mixture. To taste, add salt and pepper for seasoning.
5. Bake for 25 to 30 minutes, or until the chicken is cooked through and the skin is golden and crispy, in a preheated oven.
6. Before serving, take the chicken out of the oven and rest for a few minutes.
7. If desired, garnish with freshly chopped parsley.

NUTRITIONAL INFORMATION:

(PER SERVING, ABOUT 4 SERVINGS TOTAL)
CALORIES: 320
FAT: 24G
CARBOHYDRATES: 2G
PROTEIN: 25G

CAULIFLOWER FRIED RICE WITH SHRIMP

PREP TIME: 15 MINUTES | COOK TIME: 15 MINUTES
TOTAL TIME: 30 MINUTES

INGREDIENTS:

- 1 head cauliflower, riced
- 1 lb shrimp, peeled and deveined
- 2 tablespoons sesame oil
- 2 cloves garlic, minced
- 1 small onion, diced
- 1 cup frozen mixed vegetables (peas, carrots, corn)
- 2 eggs, beaten

- 3 tablespoons soy sauce or tamari sauce
- 1 teaspoon grated ginger
- Salt and pepper to taste
- Chopped green onions for garnish (optional)
- Sesame seeds for garnish (optional)

INSTRUCTIONS:

1. In a large skillet or wok, warm the sesame oil over medium heat. Cook the chopped onion and minced garlic until tender.
2. When the shrimp are pink and opaque, add them to the skillet and simmer. Remove the shrimp from the pan and set them aside.
3. Transfer the cooked shrimp to one side of the pan and cover with the beaten eggs. Once the eggs are cooked, scramble and combine them with the onions and shrimp.
4. Add frozen mixed veggies and riced cauliflower and stir. Cook the cauliflower until it's crisp-tender.
5. Toss in the grated ginger, soy sauce (or tamari sauce), salt, and pepper. Mix everything.
6. After cooking, add the shrimp to the pan and toss to coat with sauce.
7. Cook for a further two to three minutes or until well heated.
8. Top the hot cauliflower fried rice with sesame seeds and chopped green onions if preferred.

NUTRITIONAL INFORMATION:

(PER SERVING, ABOUT 4 SERVINGS TOTAL)
CALORIES: 220
FAT: 10G
CARBOHYDRATES: 10G
PROTEIN: 20G

GREEK TURKEY MEATBALLS WITH TZATZIKI SAUCE

PREP TIME: 20 MINUTES | COOK TIME: 20 MINUTES
TOTAL TIME: 40 MINUTES

INGREDIENTS:

FOR THE MEATBALLS:

- 1 lb ground turkey
- 1/4 cup breadcrumbs (or almond flour for keto)
- 1/4 cup crumbled feta cheese
- 1/4 cup chopped fresh parsley
- 1/4 cup chopped red onion
- 2 cloves garlic, minced
- 1 teaspoon dried oregano
- 1/2 teaspoon ground cumin
- Salt and pepper to taste
- Olive oil for cooking

FOR THE TZATZIKI SAUCE:

- 1 cup Greek yogurt
- 1/2 cucumber, grated and squeezed to remove excess moisture
- 1 clove garlic, minced

- 1 tablespoon chopped fresh dill
- 1 tablespoon lemon juice
- Salt and pepper to taste

INSTRUCTIONS:

1. Set oven temperature to 400°F or 200°C. Use parchment paper to line a baking sheet.
2. Ground turkey, breadcrumbs (or almond flour), crumbled feta cheese, minced garlic, chopped red onion, chopped parsley, ground cumin, dried oregano, and salt and pepper should all be combined in a big mixing basin. Blend until well blended.
3. Form the turkey mixture into meatballs and arrange them on the baking sheet that has been preheated.
4. Coat the meatballs with olive oil and bake in the oven for 18 to 20 minutes or until they are cooked through and have a browned exterior.
5. Make the tzatziki sauce while the meatballs are baking. Combine Greek yogurt, grated cucumber, minced garlic, chopped dill, lemon juice, salt, and pepper in a bowl. Blend until well blended.
6. Serve the tzatziki sauce beside the hot Greek turkey meatballs.

NUTRITIONAL INFORMATION:

(PER SERVING, ABOUT 4 SERVINGS TOTAL)
CALORIES: 280
FAT: 15G
CARBOHYDRATES: 7G
PROTEIN: 25G

COCONUT CURRY SALMON WITH CAULIFLOWER RICE

PREP TIME: 15 MINUTES | COOK TIME: 20 MINUTES
TOTAL TIME: 35 MINUTES

INGREDIENTS:

- 4 salmon fillets
- 2 tablespoons coconut oil
- 1 small onion, diced
- 2 cloves garlic, minced
- 1 tablespoon grated ginger
- 2 tablespoons red curry paste
- 1 (14 oz) can coconut milk
- 2 cups cauliflower rice
- Salt and pepper to taste
- Chopped fresh cilantro for garnish (optional)
- Lime wedges for serving

INSTRUCTIONS:

1. To taste, add salt and pepper to the salmon fillets.
2. Warm the coconut oil in a large pan set over medium heat. Add the grated ginger, minced garlic, and chopped onion. Simmer until aromatic and tender.
3. Add the red curry paste and let it simmer for a minute or two.
4. After adding the coconut milk, boil the mixture.

5. Place the skin-side-down salmon fillets in the skillet. After 5 to 7 minutes of cooking under cover, the salmon should flake easily with a fork and be cooked through.
6. In the meanwhile, preheat another skillet over medium heat. Cook the cauliflower rice until it becomes soft.
7. Warm coconut curry fish should be served with cauliflower rice.
8. Add finely chopped fresh cilantro as a garnish and present the salmon with lime wedges for you to squeeze over it.

NUTRITIONAL INFORMATION:
(PER SERVING, ABOUT 4 SERVINGS TOTAL)
CALORIES: 350
FAT: 25G
CARBOHYDRATES: 6G
PROTEIN: 30G

BEEF AND CAULIFLOWER SKILLET HASH
PREP TIME: 10 MINUTES | COOK TIME: 20 MINUTES
TOTAL TIME: 30 MINUTES

INGREDIENTS:
- 1 lb ground beef
- 1 small onion, diced
- 2 cloves garlic, minced
- 1 medium-head cauliflower, cut into small florets
- 1 bell pepper, diced
- 1 teaspoon paprika
- 1/2 teaspoon cumin
- Salt and pepper to taste
- Chopped fresh parsley for garnish (optional)

INSTRUCTIONS:
1. Brown the ground beef in a large pan over medium heat. While leaving the fat in the pan, remove the steak and put it aside.
2. To the skillet, add the minced garlic and chopped onion. Simmer until aromatic and tender.
3. Add the chopped bell pepper and cauliflower florets to the pan. Sauté the veggies until they are soft.
4. The cooked ground beef should be added back to the skillet. Add cumin and paprika and stir. To taste, add salt and pepper for seasoning.
5. Stirring regularly, cook for five minutes or until everything is well cooked and well blended.
6. Top the hot beef and cauliflower skillet hash with finely chopped fresh parsley if preferred.

NUTRITIONAL INFORMATION:
(PER SERVING, ABOUT 4 SERVINGS TOTAL)
CALORIES: 280
FAT: 18G
CARBOHYDRATES: 8G
PROTEIN: 24G

CREAMY GARLIC PARMESAN CHICKEN THIGHS

PREP TIME: 10 MINUTES | COOK TIME: 25 MINUTES
TOTAL TIME: 35 MINUTES

INGREDIENTS:
- 4 bone-in, skin-on chicken thighs
- Salt and pepper to taste
- 2 tablespoons butter
- 4 cloves garlic, minced
- 1 cup chicken broth
- 1/2 cup heavy cream
- 1/4 cup grated Parmesan cheese
- Chopped fresh parsley for garnish (optional)

INSTRUCTIONS:
1. On both sides, season chicken thighs with salt and pepper.
2. Melt butter in a big skillet over medium heat. Place the chicken thighs skin-side down and cook for approximately 5 minutes on each side, or until golden brown. Remove the chicken from the skillet and set it aside.
3. Add the minced garlic to the same skillet and heat until aromatic.
4. After adding chicken stock to the skillet, boil it while scraping off any browned pieces from the pan's bottom.
5. Add grated Parmesan cheese and heavy cream, and stir. Simmer until the sauce begins to slightly thicken.
6. Spoon some sauce over the chicken thighs when you put them back in the pan.
7. When the chicken is cooked through and reaches an internal temperature of 165°F (75°C), cover and boil it for 15 to 20 minutes.
8. Before serving, sprinkle some freshly chopped parsley on top.

NUTRITIONAL INFORMATION:
(PER SERVING, ABOUT 4 SERVINGS TOTAL)
CALORIES: 380
FAT: 28G
CARBOHYDRATES: 2G
PROTEIN: 30G

MEXICAN CAULIFLOWER RICE BOWL

PREP TIME: 10 MINUTES | COOK TIME: 15 MINUTES
TOTAL TIME: 25 MINUTES

INGREDIENTS:
- 1 medium head cauliflower, riced
- 1 tablespoon olive oil
- 1 small onion, diced
- 1 bell pepper, diced
- 1 cup cooked black beans
- 1 cup corn kernels (fresh, canned, or frozen)

- 1 teaspoon chilli powder
- 1/2 teaspoon cumin
- Salt and pepper to taste
- Sliced avocado, chopped cilantro, and lime wedges for serving

INSTRUCTIONS:

1. Heat the olive oil in a big skillet over medium heat. Add the bell pepper and chopped onion. Simmer until tender.
2. Add the cooked black beans, corn kernels, and riced cauliflower and stir. Cook the cauliflower until it's crisp-tender.
3. Add salt, pepper, cumin, and chilli powder to taste. Mix everything.
4. Cook for a further two to three minutes or until well heated.
5. Top the hot Mexican cauliflower rice dish with lime wedges, chopped cilantro, and sliced avocado.

NUTRITIONAL INFORMATION:

(PER SERVING, ABOUT 4 SERVINGS TOTAL)
CALORIES: 180
FAT: 6G
CARBOHYDRATES: 28G
PROTEIN: 7G

TERIYAKI TOFU STIR-FRY WITH BROCCOLI

PREP TIME: 15 MINUTES | COOK TIME: 15 MINUTES
TOTAL TIME: 30 MINUTES

INGREDIENTS:

- 1 block (14 oz) firm tofu, pressed and cubed
- 2 tablespoons cornstarch
- 2 tablespoons soy sauce
- 1 tablespoon sesame oil
- 1 tablespoon honey or maple syrup
- 2 cloves garlic, minced
- 1 teaspoon grated ginger
- 2 cups broccoli florets
- Cooked rice for serving
- Sliced green onions and sesame seeds for garnish (optional)

INSTRUCTIONS:

1. Coat the cubed tofu equally with cornstarch by tossing it in a basin.
2. To create the teriyaki sauce, combine the soy sauce, sesame oil, honey (or maple syrup), chopped garlic, and grated ginger in a separate bowl.
3. Turn the heat up to medium-high in a skillet or wok. Add the tofu cubes and fry them until they are crispy and golden brown. Remove the tofu from the pan and set it aside.
4. Add the broccoli florets and a little water to the same skillet. Once the broccoli is tender, simmer it covered.
5. Put the cooked tofu back in the skillet. Cover the tofu and broccoli with the teriyaki sauce.
6. Stirring regularly, cook for two to three more minutes, or until everything is well cooked and covered with sauce.

7. Turn the prepared rice into a bed of hot teriyaki tofu stir-fry.
8. If preferred, garnish with sesame seeds and sliced green onions.

NUTRITIONAL INFORMATION:

(PER SERVING, ABOUT 4 SERVINGS TOTAL)
CALORIES: 250
FAT: 10G
CARBOHYDRATES: 25G
PROTEIN: 15G

PORK TENDERLOIN WITH DIJON MUSTARD SAUCE

PREP TIME: 10 MINUTES | COOK TIME: 25 MINUTES
TOTAL TIME: 35 MINUTES

INGREDIENTS:

- 1 lb pork tenderloin
- Salt and pepper to taste
- 2 tablespoons olive oil
- 2 cloves garlic, minced
- 1/2 cup chicken broth
- 2 tablespoons Dijon mustard
- 1 tablespoon honey or maple syrup
- 1 tablespoon balsamic vinegar
- Chopped fresh parsley for garnish (optional)

INSTRUCTIONS:

1. Set oven temperature to 400°F or 200°C.
2. Pork tenderloin should be seasoned on both sides with salt & pepper.
3. Heat the olive oil in an ovenproof skillet over medium-high heat. When aromatic, add the minced garlic and simmer.
4. Sear the pork tenderloin in the skillet until it becomes golden brown on both sides.
5. Place the pan in the warmed oven, and roast the pig for 15 to 20 minutes, or until its internal temperature reaches 145°F (63°C).
6. Place the pork tenderloin on a chopping board after taking the pan out of the oven. Before slicing, let it a few minutes to rest.
7. Return the skillet to the burner and turn the heat down to medium. Add the chicken stock, balsamic vinegar, honey (or maple syrup), and Dijon mustard to the pan. Simmer for a little while, or until the sauce begins to thicken slightly.
8. Once the pork tenderloin is sliced, sprinkle it with the Dijon mustard sauce and serve it hot. If desired, garnish with freshly chopped parsley.

NUTRITIONAL INFORMATION:

(PER SERVING, ABOUT 4 SERVINGS TOTAL)
CALORIES: 250
FAT: 10G
CARBOHYDRATES: 5G
PROTEIN: 30G

CHICKEN ALFREDO WITH ZUCCHINI NOODLES

PREP TIME: 15 MINUTES | COOK TIME: 15 MINUTES
TOTAL TIME: 30 MINUTES

INGREDIENTS:

- 2 boneless, skinless chicken breasts, thinly sliced
- Salt and pepper to taste
- 2 tablespoons olive oil
- 3 cloves garlic, minced
- 1 cup heavy cream
- 1/2 cup grated Parmesan cheese
- 2 medium zucchini, spiralized into noodles
- Chopped fresh parsley for garnish (optional)

INSTRUCTIONS:

1. Add salt and pepper to thinly cut chicken breasts.
2. Warm the olive oil in a large skillet set over medium-high heat. Add the chicken slices and cook thoroughly until golden brown. Remove the chicken from the skillet and set it aside.
3. Add the minced garlic to the same skillet and heat until aromatic.
4. Add heavy cream to the pan and heat until it begins to boil. Simmer until the sauce begins to slightly thicken.
5. Add the grated Parmesan cheese and stir until it melts and blends well.
6. Spiralized zucchini noodles should be added to the pan and tossed to coat with Alfredo sauce. Sauté the zucchini noodles for 2 to 3 minutes or until they are crisp-tender.
7. Bring the cooked chicken back to the pan and mix it with the zucchini noodles and Alfredo sauce.
8. Top the heated zucchini noodles with chopped fresh parsley and serve the chicken Alfredo over them if preferred.

NUTRITIONAL INFORMATION:

(PER SERVING, ABOUT 4 SERVINGS TOTAL)
CALORIES: 350
FAT: 25G
CARBOHYDRATES: 6G
PROTEIN: 28G

SESAME GINGER BEEF STIR-FRY

PREP TIME: 20 MINUTES | COOK TIME: 10 MINUTES
TOTAL TIME: 30 MINUTES

INGREDIENTS:

- 1 lb beef sirloin, thinly sliced
- 2 tablespoons soy sauce
- 1 tablespoon sesame oil
- 2 cloves garlic, minced
- 1 tablespoon grated ginger
- 2 tablespoons olive oil
- 1 bell pepper, thinly sliced

- 1 cup snow peas
- 2 green onions, chopped
- Sesame seeds for garnish (optional)

INSTRUCTIONS:

1. Marinate thinly sliced beef sirloin for 15 to 20 minutes in a bowl with sesame oil, soy sauce, chopped garlic, and grated ginger.
2. Heat the olive oil over high heat in a large skillet or wok. Add the marinated beef pieces and fry until browned.
3. Add the snow peas and thinly sliced bell pepper to the skillet. Stir-fry the veggies for two to three minutes or until they are crisp-tender.
4. Top the stir-fry with sesame seeds and chopped green onions.
5. If preferred, serve the hot sesame ginger beef stir-fry over cauliflower rice or rice.

NUTRITIONAL INFORMATION:

(PER SERVING, ABOUT 4 SERVINGS TOTAL)
CALORIES: 280
FAT: 18G
CARBOHYDRATES: 8G
PROTEIN: 25G

CREAMY TUSCAN CHICKEN WITH SPINACH AND SUN-DRIED TOMATOES

PREP TIME: 10 MINUTES | COOK TIME: 20 MINUTES
TOTAL TIME: 30 MINUTES

INGREDIENTS:

- 4 boneless, skinless chicken breasts
- Salt and pepper to taste
- 2 tablespoons olive oil
- 3 cloves garlic, minced
- 1 cup chicken broth
- 1 cup heavy cream
- 1/2 cup grated Parmesan cheese
- 1 cup chopped spinach
- 1/2 cup chopped sun-dried tomatoes
- Chopped fresh basil for garnish (optional)

INSTRUCTIONS:

1. Season chicken breasts with salt and pepper.
2. Heat olive oil in a large skillet over medium-high heat. Add chicken breasts and cook until golden brown and cooked through. Remove chicken from skillet and set aside.
3. In the same skillet, add minced garlic and cook until fragrant.
4. Pour chicken broth into the skillet and bring to a simmer. Cook until the liquid reduces by half.
5. Stir in heavy cream and grated Parmesan cheese. Cook until the sauce thickens slightly.
6. Add chopped spinach and chopped sun-dried tomatoes to the skillet. Cook until spinach is wilted.
7. Return the cooked chicken breasts to the skillet and spoon some of the sauce over the top.

8. Cook for 2-3 minutes or until everything is heated through.
9. Serve the creamy Tuscan chicken hot, garnished with chopped fresh basil if desired.

NUTRITIONAL INFORMATION:
(PER SERVING, ABOUT 4 SERVINGS TOTAL)
CALORIES: 380
FAT: 25G
CARBOHYDRATES: 8G
PROTEIN: 30G

SPICY CAJUN SHRIMP WITH CAULIFLOWER GRITS
PREP TIME: 15 MINUTES | COOK TIME: 20 MINUTES
TOTAL TIME: 35 MINUTES

INGREDIENTS:
- 1 lb shrimp, peeled and deveined
- 2 tablespoons Cajun seasoning
- 2 tablespoons olive oil
- 1 small onion, diced
- 2 cloves garlic, minced
- 1 bell pepper, diced
- 1 cup chicken broth
- 1 head cauliflower, riced
- Salt and pepper to taste
- Chopped fresh parsley for garnish (optional)

INSTRUCTIONS:
1. In a bowl, toss peeled and deveined shrimp with Cajun seasoning until evenly coated.
2. Heat olive oil in a large skillet over medium heat. Add diced onion and minced garlic. Cook until softened and fragrant.
3. Add diced bell pepper to the skillet and cook until softened.
4. Add seasoned shrimp to the skillet and cook until pink and opaque. Remove shrimp from the skillet and set aside.
5. In the same skillet, pour chicken broth and bring to a simmer. Stir in riced cauliflower and cook until tender.
6. Season cauliflower grits with salt and pepper to taste.
7. Return cooked shrimp to the skillet and toss to combine with the cauliflower grits.
8. Serve the spicy Cajun shrimp with cauliflower grits hot, garnished with chopped fresh parsley if desired.

NUTRITIONAL INFORMATION:
(PER SERVING, ABOUT 4 SERVINGS TOTAL)
CALORIES: 250
FAT: 12G
CARBOHYDRATES: 10G
PROTEIN: 25G

BAKED COD WITH LEMON HERB BUTTER

PREP TIME: 10 MINUTES | COOK TIME: 15 MINUTES
TOTAL TIME: 25 MINUTES

INGREDIENTS:

- 4 cod fillets
- Salt and pepper to taste
- 4 tablespoons butter, melted
- Zest and juice of 1 lemon
- 2 cloves garlic, minced
- 1 tablespoon chopped fresh parsley
- 1 tablespoon chopped fresh dill
- Lemon slices for garnish (optional)

INSTRUCTIONS:

1. Preheat the oven to 400°F (200°C). Line a baking sheet with parchment paper.
2. Season cod fillets with salt and pepper on both sides. Place them on the prepared baking sheet.
3. Whisk together melted butter, lemon zest, lemon juice, minced garlic, chopped parsley, and chopped dill in a bowl.
4. Spoon the lemon herb butter mixture over the cod fillets.
5. Bake in the oven for 12-15 minutes or until the cod is opaque and flakes easily with a fork.
6. Serve the baked cod hot, garnished with lemon slices if desired.

NUTRITIONAL INFORMATION:

(PER SERVING, ABOUT 4 SERVINGS TOTAL)
CALORIES: 200
FAT: 10G
CARBOHYDRATES: 1G
PROTEIN: 25G

LOW-CARB CHICKEN FAJITA BOWL

PREP TIME: 15 MINUTES | COOK TIME: 20 MINUTES
TOTAL TIME: 35 MINUTES

INGREDIENTS:

- 1 lb chicken breasts, sliced
- 2 bell peppers, sliced
- 1 onion, sliced
- 2 tablespoons olive oil
- 1 tablespoon fajita seasoning
- Salt and pepper to taste
- Lettuce or cauliflower rice for serving
- Sliced avocado, sour cream, shredded cheese, and salsa for topping

INSTRUCTIONS:

1. In a large skillet, heat olive oil over medium-high heat. Add sliced chicken breasts and cook until browned and cooked through.

2. Remove the chicken from the skillet and set aside. In the same skillet, add sliced bell peppers and onion. Cook until softened.
3. Return the cooked chicken to the skillet. Sprinkle the fajita seasoning over the chicken and vegetables, stirring to combine.
4. Cook for 2-3 minutes, until everything is heated through and well combined.
5. Serve the chicken fajita mixture over lettuce or cauliflower rice.
6. Top with sliced avocado, sour cream, shredded cheese, and salsa.

NUTRITIONAL INFORMATION:
(PER SERVING, ABOUT 4 SERVINGS TOTAL)
CALORIES: 250
FAT: 12G
CARBOHYDRATES: 8G
PROTEIN: 25G

BEEF AND MUSHROOM SKEWERS WITH CHIMICHURRI SAUCE

PREP TIME: 15 MINUTES | COOK TIME: 10 MINUTES
TOTAL TIME: 25 MINUTES

INGREDIENTS:
- 1 lb beef sirloin, cut into cubes
- 8 oz mushrooms
- Salt and pepper to taste
- Wooden skewers soaked in water
- Chimichurri sauce for serving

CHIMICHURRI SAUCE:
- 1 cup fresh parsley leaves
- 1/4 cup fresh cilantro leaves
- 2 cloves garlic
- 1 shallot, chopped
- 1/4 cup red wine vinegar
- 1/2 cup olive oil
- Salt and pepper to taste

INSTRUCTIONS:
1. Preheat the grill to medium-high heat.
2. Season beef cubes and mushrooms with salt and pepper.
3. Thread beef cubes and mushrooms alternately onto the soaked wooden skewers.
4. Grill skewers for 3-4 minutes per side or until the beef is cooked to your desired level.
5. Meanwhile, prepare the chimichurri sauce. Combine parsley, cilantro, garlic, shallot, red wine vinegar, and olive oil in a food processor. Pulse until well combined but still slightly chunky. Season with salt and pepper to taste.
6. Serve the beef and mushroom skewers hot, with chimichurri sauce on the side.

NUTRITIONAL INFORMATION:

(PER SERVING, ABOUT 4 SERVINGS TOTAL)
CALORIES: 300
FAT: 20G
CARBOHYDRATES: 4G
PROTEIN: 25G

TURKEY AND CAULIFLOWER SHEPHERD'S PIE

PREP TIME: 20 MINUTES | COOK TIME: 30 MINUTES
TOTAL TIME: 50 MINUTES

INGREDIENTS:

- 1 lb ground turkey
- 1 onion, diced
- 2 cloves garlic, minced
- 2 cups cauliflower florets
- 1 cup beef or chicken broth
- 1 cup frozen mixed vegetables
- 2 tablespoons tomato paste
- Salt and pepper to taste
- Mashed cauliflower for topping
- Chopped fresh parsley for garnish (optional)

INSTRUCTIONS:

1. Preheat oven to 375°F (190°C).
2. In a skillet, cook ground turkey, diced onion, and minced garlic until turkey is browned and cooked through.
3. Steam cauliflower florets until tender. Mash them with a fork or potato masher.
4. Add beef or chicken broth, frozen mixed vegetables, and tomato paste to the skillet with the cooked turkey. Season with salt and pepper to taste. Cook until heated through and slightly thickened.
5. Transfer the turkey mixture to a baking dish. Spread mashed cauliflower over the top.
6. Bake in the preheated oven for 25-30 minutes or until the top is golden brown.
7. Garnish with chopped fresh parsley before serving.

NUTRITIONAL INFORMATION:

(PER SERVING, ABOUT 4 SERVINGS TOTAL)
CALORIES: 280
FAT: 10G
CARBOHYDRATES: 12G
PROTEIN: 25G

LEMON GARLIC BUTTER SHRIMP SCAMPI

PREP TIME: 10 MINUTES | COOK TIME: 10 MINUTES
TOTAL TIME: 20 MINUTES

INGREDIENTS:

- 1 lb shrimp, peeled and deveined
- Salt and pepper to taste
- 2 tablespoons olive oil
- 4 cloves garlic, minced
- Zest and juice of 1 lemon
- 2 tablespoons butter
- Chopped fresh parsley for garnish (optional)

INSTRUCTIONS:

1. Season shrimp with salt and pepper.
2. Heat olive oil in a large skillet over medium heat. Add minced garlic and cook until fragrant.
3. Add shrimp to the skillet and cook until pink and opaque.
4. Stir in lemon zest, lemon juice, and butter. Cook until the butter is melted and the shrimp are coated in the sauce.
5. Serve the lemon garlic butter shrimp scampi hot, garnished with chopped fresh parsley if desired.

NUTRITIONAL INFORMATION:

(PER SERVING, ABOUT 4 SERVINGS TOTAL)
CALORIES: 200
FAT: 10G
CARBOHYDRATES: 2G
PROTEIN: 25G

THAI BASIL CHICKEN STIR-FRY

PREP TIME: 15 MINUTES | COOK TIME: 10 MINUTES
TOTAL TIME: 25 MINUTES

INGREDIENTS:

- 1 lb chicken breasts, thinly sliced
- Salt and pepper to taste
- 2 tablespoons vegetable oil
- 3 cloves garlic, minced
- 1 red bell pepper, thinly sliced
- 1 onion, thinly sliced
- 2 tablespoons oyster sauce
- 1 tablespoon soy sauce
- 1 tablespoon fish sauce
- 1 tablespoon sugar or sweetener
- 1 cup fresh basil leaves
- Cooked rice for serving

INSTRUCTIONS:

1. Season thinly sliced chicken breasts with salt and pepper.
2. Heat vegetable oil in a large skillet or wok over high heat. Add minced garlic and cook until fragrant.
3. Add sliced chicken to the skillet and stir-fry until browned and cooked through.
4. Add thinly sliced red bell pepper and onion to the skillet. Stir-fry until vegetables are tender.
5. Mix oyster sauce, soy sauce, fish sauce, and sugar or sweetener in a small bowl. Pour the sauce over the chicken and vegetables.
6. Stir in fresh basil leaves and cook until wilted.
7. Serve the Thai basil chicken stir-fry hot, overcooked rice.

NUTRITIONAL INFORMATION:
(PER SERVING, ABOUT 4 SERVINGS TOTAL)
CALORIES: 280
FAT: 15G
CARBOHYDRATES: 8G
PROTEIN: 25G

KETO BBQ RIBS WITH COLESLAW

PREP TIME: 15 MINUTES | COOK TIME: 3 HOURS
TOTAL TIME: 3 HOURS 15 MINUTES

INGREDIENTS:
- 2 racks of pork ribs
- Salt and pepper to taste
- 1 cup sugar-free barbecue sauce
- 1/4 cup apple cider vinegar
- 1 tablespoon Worcestershire sauce
- 1 tablespoon smoked paprika
- 1 tablespoon garlic powder
- 1 tablespoon onion powder
- 1 tablespoon chilli powder
- 1 teaspoon liquid smoke (optional)
- Coleslaw for serving

INSTRUCTIONS:
1. Turn the oven on to 300°F or 150°C.
2. Use salt and pepper to season the pork ribs. Tightly encase each rack with aluminium foil.
3. Once the oven is ready, place the foil-wrapped ribs on a baking sheet and bake for 2.5–3 hours or until they are tender.
4. Combine sugar-free barbecue sauce, Worcestershire sauce, apple cider vinegar, smoked paprika, garlic powder, onion powder, chili powder, and liquid smoke in a bowl, if desired.
5. After taking the ribs out of the oven, gently unwrap them. Apply a liberal amount of the barbecue sauce mixture on the ribs.
6. Grill at a medium-high temperature. Brush the ribs with more barbecue sauce and grill for ten to fifteen minutes or until they are caramelized and gently browned.
7. Warm up the keto BBQ ribs and serve them with a side of coleslaw.

NUTRITIONAL INFORMATION:
(PER SERVING, ABOUT 4 SERVINGS TOTAL)

CALORIES: 400
FAT: 30G
CARBOHYDRATES: 5G
PROTEIN: 25G

EGGPLANT PARMESAN WITH MARINARA SAUCE

PREP TIME: 20 MINUTES | COOK TIME: 40 MINUTES
TOTAL TIME: 1 HOUR

INGREDIENTS:

- 2 medium eggplants, sliced into rounds
- Salt
- 1 cup almond flour
- 2 eggs, beaten
- 1 cup grated Parmesan cheese
- 2 cups marinara sauce
- 1 cup shredded mozzarella cheese
- Fresh basil leaves for garnish (optional)

INSTRUCTIONS:

1. Turn the oven on to 375°F, or 190°C. Coat a baking sheet with oil.
2. Arrange the eggplant rounds on a baking sheet covered with paper towels. To extract moisture, sprinkle with salt and let it for fifteen minutes.
3. Using paper towels, pat the slices of eggplant dry.
4. Combine almond flour, beaten eggs, and grated Parmesan cheese in separate shallow dishes.
5. Coat each eggplant slice uniformly by dipping it first in almond flour, then in beaten eggs, and lastly in grated Parmesan cheese.
6. Arrange the coated eggplant slices on the prepared baking sheet. Bake in a preheated oven for 20 to 25 minutes, or until crispy and golden brown.
7. Take the slices of eggplant out of the oven. Drizzle each slice with marinara sauce and top with mozzarella cheese shreds.
8. Place the baking sheet back in the oven and continue baking for fifteen minutes or until the cheese is bubbling and melted.
9. Before serving, garnish with fresh basil leaves.

NUTRITIONAL INFORMATION:

(PER SERVING, ABOUT 6 SERVINGS TOTAL)
CALORIES: 250
FAT: 15G
CARBOHYDRATES: 10G
PROTEIN: 15G

GRILLED LEMON HERB CHICKEN BREASTS

PREP TIME: 10 MINUTES | COOK TIME: 15 MINUTES
TOTAL TIME: 25 MINUTES

INGREDIENTS:

- 4 boneless, skinless chicken breasts
- Salt and pepper to taste
- 2 tablespoons olive oil
- Zest and juice of 1 lemon
- 2 cloves garlic, minced
- 1 tablespoon chopped fresh parsley
- 1 tablespoon chopped fresh thyme
- Lemon slices for garnish (optional)

INSTRUCTIONS:

1. Grill at a medium-high temperature.
2. Add salt and pepper to chicken breasts for seasoning.
3. Olive oil, lemon zest, lemon juice, minced garlic, chopped parsley, and chopped thyme should all be combined in a bowl.
4. Drizzle the chicken breasts with a combination of lemon and herbs.
5. Chicken breasts should be cooked through and no longer pink in the middle after grilling them for 6–7 minutes on each side.
6. If desired, top the hot grilled lemon-herb chicken breasts with sliced lemons.

NUTRITIONAL INFORMATION:

(PER SERVING, ABOUT 4 SERVINGS TOTAL)
CALORIES: 250
FAT: 10G
CARBOHYDRATES: 0G
PROTEIN: 35G

MOROCCAN SPICED LAMB CHOPS WITH CAULIFLOWER COUSCOUS

PREP TIME: 15 MINUTES | COOK TIME: 15 MINUTES
TOTAL TIME: 30 MINUTES

INGREDIENTS:

- 4 lamb chops
- 2 teaspoons ground cumin
- 1 teaspoon ground coriander
- 1 teaspoon paprika
- 1/2 teaspoon ground cinnamon
- Salt and pepper to taste

- 2 tablespoons olive oil
- 1 head cauliflower, grated or processed into a couscous-like texture
- 1/4 cup chopped fresh parsley
- 1/4 cup chopped fresh mint
- Juice of 1 lemon

INSTRUCTIONS:

1. Combine the ground cumin, coriander, cinnamon, paprika, salt, and pepper in a small bowl.
2. Make sure the lamb chops are uniformly covered by rubbing them with the spice mixture.
3. Warm the olive oil in a pan set over medium-high heat. Add the lamb chops and fry for 3–4 minutes on each side until browned and cooked to your preferred doneness.
4. Make the cauliflower couscous while the lamb chops are cooking. Heat a tablespoon of olive oil in a different skillet over medium heat. Add the grated cauliflower and simmer, stirring regularly, for 5 to 6 minutes or until tender.
5. Take the cauliflower couscous off the stove and mix in the lemon juice, chopped fresh mint, and chopped fresh parsley.
6. Warm lamb chops marinated in Moroccan spices should be served with cauliflower couscous.

NUTRITIONAL INFORMATION:

(PER SERVING, ABOUT 4 SERVINGS TOTAL)
CALORIES: 350
FAT: 20G
CARBOHYDRATES: 10G
PROTEIN: 30G

COCONUT LIME SHRIMP WITH CAULIFLOWER RICE

PREP TIME: 10 MINUTES | COOK TIME: 10 MINUTES
TOTAL TIME: 20 MINUTES

INGREDIENTS:

- 1 lb shrimp, peeled and deveined
- Salt and pepper to taste
- 2 tablespoons coconut oil
- 3 cloves garlic, minced
- Zest and juice of 1 lime
- 1/4 cup coconut milk
- 1 head cauliflower, grated or processed into rice-like texture
- Chopped fresh cilantro for garnish (optional)

INSTRUCTIONS:

1. Add some salt and pepper to the shrimp.
2. In a pan over medium heat, preheat the coconut oil. When aromatic, add the minced garlic and simmer.
3. Cook the shrimp in the pan for two to three minutes on each side or until they are opaque and pink.
4. Add the coconut milk, lime juice, and zest. Simmer for one or two more minutes.
5. Make the cauliflower rice while the shrimp are cooking. In a separate pan, heat one tablespoon of coconut oil over medium heat. When the cauliflower is cooked, add the grated cauliflower and simmer, stirring periodically, for 4–5 minutes.

6. Over cauliflower rice, serve the hot coconut lime shrimp.
7. If desired, garnish with freshly cut cilantro.

NUTRITIONAL INFORMATION:
(PER SERVING, ABOUT 4 SERVINGS TOTAL)
CALORIES: 250
FAT: 15G
CARBOHYDRATES: 10G
PROTEIN: 20G

BEEF AND CABBAGE STIR-FRY
PREP TIME: 15 MINUTES | COOK TIME: 15 MINUTES
TOTAL TIME: 30 MINUTES

INGREDIENTS:
- 1 lb beef sirloin, thinly sliced
- 2 tablespoons soy sauce
- 1 tablespoon sesame oil
- 1 tablespoon olive oil
- 3 cloves garlic, minced
- 1 onion, thinly sliced
- 1/2 head cabbage, thinly sliced
- Salt and pepper to taste
- Chopped green onions for garnish (optional)

INSTRUCTIONS:
1. Thinly slice the beef sirloin and marinate it in sesame oil and soy sauce for ten to fifteen minutes.
2. Heat the olive oil over high heat in a large skillet or wok. When aromatic, add the minced garlic and simmer.
3. Stir-fry the marinated beef pieces in the pan until they are browned.
4. To the skillet, add the thinly sliced onion and cabbage. Add the veggies and stir-fry until soft.
5. To taste, add salt and pepper for seasoning.
6. Serve the hot stir-fried beef and cabbage with chopped green onions on top, if preferred.

NUTRITIONAL INFORMATION:
(PER SERVING, ABOUT 4 SERVINGS TOTAL)
CALORIES: 300
FAT: 15G
CARBOHYDRATES: 10G
PROTEIN: 25G

STUFFED CHICKEN BREAST WITH SPINACH AND FETA

PREP TIME: 20 MINUTES | COOK TIME: 25 MINUTES
TOTAL TIME: 45 MINUTES

INGREDIENTS:

- 4 boneless, skinless chicken breasts
- Salt and pepper to taste
- 2 cups baby spinach
- 1/2 cup crumbled feta cheese
- 2 cloves garlic, minced
- 1 tablespoon olive oil
- Toothpicks or kitchen twine

INSTRUCTIONS:

1. Turn the oven on to 375°F, or 190°C. Coat a baking dish with oil.
2. Add salt and pepper to the chicken breasts for seasoning. With a sharp knife, cut a pocket into the side of each chicken breast.
3. Heat the olive oil in a pan over medium heat. When aromatic, add the minced garlic and simmer.
4. Cook the young spinach in the skillet until it wilts.
5. Take the pan off of the burner and add the crumbled feta cheese.
6. Stuff the spinach and feta mixture inside each chicken breast. If necessary, fasten with toothpicks or kitchen thread.
7. Stuff the chicken breasts into the prepared baking dish. Bake in a preheated oven for 20 to 25 minutes, or until the chicken is well cooked.
8. Before serving, take off the kitchen twine or toothpicks.

NUTRITIONAL INFORMATION:

(PER SERVING, ABOUT 4 SERVINGS TOTAL)
CALORIES: 300
FAT: 15G
CARBOHYDRATES: 2G
PROTEIN: 35G

BAKED PESTO CHICKEN WITH CHERRY TOMATOES

PREP TIME: 10 MINUTES | COOK TIME: 25 MINUTES
TOTAL TIME: 35 MINUTES

INGREDIENTS:

- 4 boneless, skinless chicken breasts
- Salt and pepper to taste
- 1/4 cup pesto sauce
- 1 cup cherry tomatoes, halved
- 1/4 cup grated Parmesan cheese
- Chopped fresh basil for garnish (optional)

INSTRUCTIONS:

1. Turn the oven on to 375°F, or 190°C. Coat a baking dish with oil.
2. Add salt and pepper to chicken breasts for seasoning. Put them in the baking dish that has been prepared.
3. Evenly cover each chicken breast with pesto sauce.
4. Halve the cherry tomatoes and distribute them over the chicken breasts.
5. Over the chicken and tomatoes, scatter the grated Parmesan cheese.
6. Bake in a preheated oven for 20 to 25 minutes, or until the chicken is well cooked.
7. Before serving, garnish with finely chopped fresh basil.

NUTRITIONAL INFORMATION:

(PER SERVING, ABOUT 4 SERVINGS TOTAL)
CALORIES: 250
FAT: 15G
CARBOHYDRATES: 3G
PROTEIN: 30G

SPICY TOFU AND VEGETABLE STIR-FRY

PREP TIME: 15 MINUTES | COOK TIME: 15 MINUTES
TOTAL TIME: 30 MINUTES

INGREDIENTS:
- 1 block extra-firm tofu, pressed and cubed
- 2 tablespoons soy sauce
- 1 tablespoon sesame oil
- 1 tablespoon olive oil
- 3 cloves garlic, minced
- 1 red bell pepper, thinly sliced
- 1 green bell pepper, thinly sliced
- 1 cup snap peas
- 2 green onions, chopped
- 1 tablespoon Sriracha sauce (adjust to taste)
- Salt and pepper to taste

INSTRUCTIONS:
1. Marinate cubed tofu in a dish with sesame oil and soy sauce

 for ten to fifteen minutes.

2. Heat the olive oil over high heat in a large skillet or wok. When aromatic, add the minced garlic and simmer.
3. Stir-fry the marinated tofu pieces in the pan until they become golden brown.
4. The pan should be filled with snap peas, chopped green onions, thinly sliced red and green bell peppers, and snap peas. Add the veggies and stir-fry until soft.
5. Add the Sriracha sauce, taste, and adjust the seasoning with salt and pepper.
6. Serve the hot, spicy, stir-fried tofu and vegetables over cooked or cauliflower rice.

NUTRITIONAL INFORMATION:
(PER SERVING, ABOUT 4 SERVINGS TOTAL)
CALORIES: 200
FAT: 10G
CARBOHYDRATES: 10G
PROTEIN: 15G

LEMON HERB GRILLED PORK CHOPS

PREP TIME: 10 MINUTES | COOK TIME: 15 MINUTES
TOTAL TIME: 25 MINUTES

INGREDIENTS:

- 4 bone-in pork chops
- Salt and pepper to taste
- Zest and juice of 1 lemon
- 2 cloves garlic, minced
- 1 tablespoon chopped fresh rosemary
- 1 tablespoon chopped fresh thyme
- 2 tablespoons olive oil

INSTRUCTIONS:

1. Use salt and pepper to season the pork chops.
2. Combine the lemon zest, lemon juice, olive oil, minced garlic, chopped fresh rosemary, chopped fresh thyme, and chopped fresh rosemary in a small bowl.
3. Ensure the pork chops are uniformly covered by rubbing them with the lemon herb mixture.
4. Grill at a medium-high temperature. Pork chops should be cooked through and no longer pink in the middle after grilling them for 6–7 minutes on each side.
5. Serve the hot grilled pork chops with lemon and herbs.

NUTRITIONAL INFORMATION:

(PER SERVING, ABOUT 4 SERVINGS TOTAL)
CALORIES: 300
FAT: 20G
CARBOHYDRATES: 0G
PROTEIN: 30G

KETO CHOCOLATE AVOCADO MOUSSE

PREP TIME: 10 MINUTES | COOK TIME: 0 MINUTES
TOTAL TIME: 10 MINUTES

INGREDIENTS:

- 2 ripe avocados
- 1/4 cup unsweetened cocoa powder
- 1/4 cup powdered erythritol or sweetener of choice
- 1 teaspoon vanilla extract
- Pinch of salt
- 1/4 cup unsweetened almond milk or coconut milk (optional, for desired consistency)

INSTRUCTIONS:

1. Halve the avocados and scoop out the pits. Remove the avocado flesh and place it in a food processor or blender.
2. Adddd vanilla extract, cocoa powder, powdered erythritol, and a sprinkle of in a blender or food processor salt.
3. Scrape down the sides as necessary, and blend until creamy and smooth.
4. If the mousse is too thick, add almond or coconut milk a tablespoon at a time until it reaches the right consistency.
5. Spoon the mousse into glasses or serving dishes.
6. Let it cool for a minimum of half an hour before serving.
7. Before serving, add whipped cream, chopped almonds, or berries as a garnish.

NUTRITIONAL INFORMATION:

(PER SERVING, ABOUT 4 SERVINGS TOTAL)
CALORIES: 200
FAT: 15G
CARBOHYDRATES: 10G
PROTEIN: 3G

LOW-CARB STRAWBERRY CHEESECAKE BITES

PREP TIME: 15 MINUTES | COOK TIME: 0 MINUTES
TOTAL TIME: 15 MINUTES

INGREDIENTS:

- 1 cup fresh strawberries, hulled
- 4 oz cream cheese, softened
- 2 tablespoons powdered erythritol or sweetener of choice
- 1/2 teaspoon vanilla extract
- Optional toppings: melted sugar-free chocolate, chopped nuts, shredded coconut

INSTRUCTIONS:

1. In a mixing dish, combine vanilla extract, powdered erythritol, and softened cream cheese. Blend until well combined.
2. Spoon the cream cheese mixture into each hulled strawberry using a tiny spoon or a piping bag.
3. If preferred, each stuffed strawberry may be dipped in melted sugar-free chocolate or topped with shredded coconut or chopped almonds.
4. Transfer the stuffed strawberries to a parchment paper-lined dish or tray.
5. Let it cool for a minimum of half an hour before serving.

NUTRITIONAL INFORMATION:
(PER SERVING, ABOUT 4 SERVINGS TOTAL)
CALORIES: 100
FAT: 8G
CARBOHYDRATES: 5G
PROTEIN: 2G

ALMOND FLOUR LEMON POPPY SEED CAKE
PREP TIME: 15 MINUTES | COOK TIME: 25 MINUTES
TOTAL TIME: 40 MINUTES

INGREDIENTS:
- 2 cups almond flour
- 1/3 cup erythritol or sweetener of choice
- Zest of 2 lemons
- 2 tablespoons poppy seeds
- 1 teaspoon baking powder
- 1/4 teaspoon salt
- 1/4 cup melted coconut oil or butter
- 3 large eggs
- 1/4 cup lemon juice
- 1 teaspoon vanilla extract

INSTRUCTIONS:
1. Set the oven's temperature to 175°C/350°F. An 8x8-inch baking pan may be lined with parchment paper or greased.
2. Almond flour, erythritol, poppy seeds, lemon zest, baking powder, and salt should all be combined in a mixing dish.
3. Whisk eggs, lemon juice, vanilla extract, and melted butter or coconut oil in another dish.
4. After adding the wet components to the dry ingredients, thoroughly mix them.
5. Evenly spread out the batter in the baking pan that has been prepared.
6. A toothpick put into the middle should come out clean after 20 to 25 minutes of baking in a preheated oven or until the edges are golden brown.
7. Let the cake cool fully before cutting it into slices and serving.

NUTRITIONAL INFORMATION:
(PER SERVING, ABOUT 9 SERVINGS TOTAL)
CALORIES: 200
FAT: 18G
CARBOHYDRATES: 5G

COCONUT FLOUR CHOCOLATE CHIP COOKIES

PREP TIME: 15 MINUTES | COOK TIME: 10 MINUTES
TOTAL TIME: 25 MINUTES

INGREDIENTS:

- 1/2 cup coconut flour
- 1/2 cup erythritol or sweetener of choice
- 1/4 teaspoon baking soda
- Pinch of salt
- 1/3 cup melted coconut oil
- 2 large eggs
- 1 teaspoon vanilla extract
- 1/3 cup sugar-free chocolate chips

INSTRUCTIONS:

1. Set the oven's temperature to 175°C/350°F. Use parchment paper to line a baking sheet.
2. Mix coconut flour, baking soda, erythritol, and salt in a mixing basin.
3. Whisk the eggs, vanilla extract, and melted coconut oil in another basin.
4. Mixing until a dough forms, pour the wet components into the dry ingredients.
5. Add sugar-free chocolate chips and stir.
6. Spoon or use a cookie scoop to divide out the dough and transfer it to the ready baking sheet.
7. Using your hands, gently flatten each biscuit.
8. Bake in a preheated oven for 8 to 10 minutes, or until the edges are golden brown.
9. After a few minutes of cooling on the baking sheet, move the cookies to a wire rack to finish cooling.

NUTRITIONAL INFORMATION:

(PER SERVING, ABOUT 12 SERVINGS TOTAL)
CALORIES: 150
FAT: 12G
CARBOHYDRATES: 5G
PROTEIN: 3G

SUGAR-FREE BLUEBERRY CHIA SEED PUDDING

PREP TIME: 5 MINUTES | COOK TIME: 0 MINUTES
TOTAL TIME: 5 MINUTES (PLUS CHILLING TIME)

INGREDIENTS:

- 1 cup unsweetened almond milk or coconut milk
- 1/4 cup chia seeds
- 1 tablespoon powdered erythritol or sweetener of choice
- 1/2 teaspoon vanilla extract
- 1/2 cup fresh or frozen blueberries

INSTRUCTIONS:

1. Mix the powdered erythritol, chia seeds, almond milk, and vanilla essence in a jar or dish.
2. Add frozen or fresh blueberries and stir.
3. Once the chia pudding has thickened, cover the dish or jar and place it in the refrigerator for at least two hours or overnight.
4. Before serving, stir the pudding and, if required, thin it with more almond milk.
5. Serve cold, with the option to add more blueberries or any desired toppings.

NUTRITIONAL INFORMATION:
(PER SERVING, ABOUT 2 SERVINGS TOTAL)
CALORIES: 100
FAT: 6G
CARBOHYDRATES: 8G
PROTEIN: 3G

CHOCOLATE PEANUT BUTTER FAT BOMBS
PREP TIME: 10 MINUTES | COOK TIME: 0 MINUTES
TOTAL TIME: 10 MINUTES (PLUS CHILLING TIME)

INGREDIENTS:
- 1/2 cup coconut oil, melted
- 1/4 cup unsweetened cocoa powder
- 1/4 cup powdered erythritol or sweetener of choice
- 1/4 cup creamy peanut butter
- Pinch of salt

INSTRUCTIONS:
1. Melted coconut oil, cocoa powder, erythritol powder, creamy peanut butter, and a dash of salt should all be combined and whisked until smooth in a mixing dish.
2. Spoon mixture into tiny muffin cups or silicone candy moulds, filling each hole to nearly halfway.
3. To eliminate any air bubbles, lightly tap the muffin cups or moulds on the tabletop.
4. The fat bombs should be firmed up in the freezer after one to two hours.
5. Once solid, remove the fat bombs from the muffin tins or molds and place them in an airtight freezer or refrigerator container.

NUTRITIONAL INFORMATION:
(PER SERVING, ABOUT 8 SERVINGS TOTAL)
CALORIES: 150
FAT: 15G
CARBOHYDRATES: 3G
PROTEIN: 2G

VANILLA BEAN GREEK YOGURT PANNA COTTA

PREP TIME: 10 MINUTES | COOK TIME: 5 MINUTES
TOTAL TIME: 4 HOURS 15 MINUTES

INGREDIENTS:

- 1 cup heavy cream
- 1 cup full-fat Greek yogurt
- 1/4 cup powdered erythritol or sweetener of choice
- 1 vanilla bean, split lengthwise and seeds scraped out (or 1 teaspoon vanilla extract)
- 2 teaspoons unflavored gelatin
- 2 tablespoons cold water

INSTRUCTIONS:

1. The heavy cream, vanilla bean seeds, and powdered erythritol should be heated in a saucepan over medium heat until they barely start to boil. Take off the heat.
2. Gelatin should be sprinkled over cold water in a small basin and allowed to bloom for five minutes.
3. Whisk the bloomed gelatin into the heated cream mixture until it dissolves completely.
4. Smoothly whisk the Greek yoghurt in a different bowl.
5. Pour the heated cream mixture into the Greek yoghurt gradually while continuing to whisk until well blended.
6. Transfer the blend into serving ramekins or glasses.
7. Place in the refrigerator until firm, at least 4 hours.
8. Serve cold, with the option to top with a dollop of sugar-free syrup or fresh berries.

NUTRITIONAL INFORMATION:

(PER SERVING, ABOUT 4 SERVINGS TOTAL)
CALORIES: 200
FAT: 18G
CARBOHYDRATES: 4G
PROTEIN: 6G

RASPBERRY ALMOND FLOUR CAKE BARS

PREP TIME: 10 MINUTES | COOK TIME: 25 MINUTES
TOTAL TIME: 35 MINUTES

INGREDIENTS:

- 2 cups almond flour
- 1/4 cup coconut flour
- 1/2 cup powdered erythritol or sweetener of choice
- 1 teaspoon baking powder
- Pinch of salt
- 1/2 cup melted coconut oil or butter
- 3 large eggs
- 1/4 cup unsweetened almond milk or coconut milk

- 1 teaspoon vanilla extract
- 1 cup fresh raspberries

INSTRUCTIONS:
1. Set the oven's temperature to 175°C/350°F. Grease or use parchment paper to line a baking dish.
2. Almond flour, coconut flour, erythritol powder, baking powder, and salt should all be combined in a mixing dish.
3. Melt the butter or coconut oil, beat in the eggs, almond milk, vanilla essence, and separate bowl.
4. After adding the wet components to the dry ingredients, thoroughly mix them.
5. Add the fresh raspberries and fold.
6. Evenly spread out the batter in the baking dish that has been prepared.
7. A toothpick put into the middle should come out clean after 20 to 25 minutes of baking in a preheated oven or until the edges are golden brown.
8. Let the cake bars cool fully before cutting and arranging on a platter.

NUTRITIONAL INFORMATION:
(PER SERVING, ABOUT 12 SERVINGS TOTAL)
CALORIES: 150
FAT: 12G
CARBOHYDRATES: 5G
PROTEIN: 5G

NO-BAKE PEANUT BUTTER CHOCOLATE BARS
PREP TIME: 10 MINUTES | COOK TIME: 0 MINUTES
TOTAL TIME: 2 HOURS 10 MINUTES

INGREDIENTS:
- 1 cup creamy peanut butter
- 1/4 cup coconut oil, melted
- 1/4 cup powdered erythritol or sweetener of choice
- 1 teaspoon vanilla extract
- 2 cups almond flour
- 1/2 cup sugar-free chocolate chips

INSTRUCTIONS:
1. Grease an 8 × 8-inch baking dish with cooking parchment.
2. Put the powdered erythritol, heated coconut oil, vanilla extract, and creamy peanut butter in a mixing dish. Blend until well combined.
3. Add almond flour gradually and whisk until well mixed.
4. Evenly press the mixture into the bottom of the baking dish that has been prepared.
5. Use a double boiler or the microwave to melt sugar-free chocolate chips.
6. Evenly distribute the melted chocolate over the peanut butter mixture after pouring it on top.
7. Place in the refrigerator until solid, at least 2 hours.
8. Cut into bars and serve once firm.

NUTRITIONAL INFORMATION:
(PER SERVING, ABOUT 16 SERVINGS TOTAL)
CALORIES: 200

FAT: 18G
CARBOHYDRATES: 5G
PROTEIN: 6G

KETO COCONUT MACAROONS

PREP TIME: 10 MINUTES | COOK TIME: 15 MINUTES
TOTAL TIME: 25 MINUTES

INGREDIENTS:

- 2 cups unsweetened shredded coconut
- 1/2 cup powdered erythritol or sweetener of choice
- 2 large egg whites
- 1/2 teaspoon vanilla extract
- Pinch of salt

INSTRUCTIONS:

1. Set oven temperature to 325°F, or 160°C. Use parchment paper to line a baking sheet.
2. Put powdered erythritol and unsweetened shredded coconut in a mixing dish.
3. Lightly whisk egg whites in another bowl until frothy.
4. Add a little teaspoon of salt and vanilla essence to the egg whites and stir.
5. After adding the egg white mixture to the coconut mixture, thoroughly mix everything.
6. Scoop tablespoon-sized quantities of the mixture onto the prepared baking sheet using a spoon or cookie scoop.
7. Bake in a preheated oven for 12 to 15 minutes, or until the edges are golden brown.
8. After a few minutes of cooling on the baking sheet, move the coconut macaroons to a wire rack to finish cooling.

NUTRITIONAL INFORMATION:

(PER SERVING, ABOUT 12 SERVINGS TOTAL)
CALORIES: 100
FAT: 8G
CARBOHYDRATES: 5G
PROTEIN: 2G

AVOCADO CHOCOLATE FUDGE BROWNIES

PREP TIME: 15 MINUTES | COOK TIME: 25 MINUTES
TOTAL TIME: 40 MINUTES

INGREDIENTS:

- 2 ripe avocados
- 1/2 cup unsweetened cocoa powder
- 1/2 cup powdered erythritol or sweetener of choice
- 2 large eggs
- 1 teaspoon vanilla extract
- 1/4 cup almond flour
- 1/4 teaspoon baking powder

- Pinch of salt
- 1/2 cup sugar-free chocolate chips

INSTRUCTIONS:

1. Set the oven's temperature to 175°C/350°F. Grease or use parchment paper to line a baking dish.
2. Mash the ripe avocados until smooth in a mixing dish.
3. Add the powdered erythritol and unsweetened cocoa powder and stir until well-mixed.
4. Blend in eggs and vanilla essence until well combined.
5. Mix baking powder, almond flour, and a little salt in another basin.
6. Mixing until well blended, gradually add the dry ingredients to the wet components.
7. Add sugar-free chocolate chips and stir.
8. Evenly distribute the batter after pouring it into the ready baking dish.
9. Bake in the preheated oven for 20 to 25 minutes, or until a toothpick inserted in the middle comes out largely clean.
10. Let cool fully before slicing and serving the brownies.

NUTRITIONAL INFORMATION:

(PER SERVING, ABOUT 12 SERVINGS TOTAL)
CALORIES: 150
FAT: 12G
CARBOHYDRATES: 7G
PROTEIN: 3G

LEMON RICOTTA CHEESECAKE MUFFINS

PREP TIME: 15 MINUTES | COOK TIME: 25 MINUTES
TOTAL TIME: 40 MINUTES

INGREDIENTS:

- 1 cup almond flour
- 1/4 cup coconut flour
- 1/2 cup powdered erythritol or sweetener of choice
- 1 teaspoon baking powder
- Pinch of salt
- 1/4 cup melted coconut oil or butter
- 3 large eggs
- 1/4 cup ricotta cheese
- Zest and juice of 1 lemon
- 1 teaspoon vanilla extract

INSTRUCTIONS:

1. Set the oven's temperature to 175°C/350°F. Use paper liners to line a muffin tray.
2. Almond flour, coconut flour, erythritol powder, baking powder, and salt should all be combined in a mixing dish.
3. Melted butter or coconut oil, eggs, ricotta cheese, lemon zest, lemon juice, and vanilla essence should all be combined in a different bowl.
4. After adding the wet components to the dry ingredients, thoroughly mix them.
5. Evenly distribute the batter among the muffin tins.
6. Bake for 20 to 25 minutes or until the tops of the muffins are firm and browned.
7. After five minutes of cooling in the muffin tray, move the muffins to a wire rack to finish cooling.

NUTRITIONAL INFORMATION:

(PER SERVING, ABOUT 12 SERVINGS TOTAL)
CALORIES: 150
FAT: 12G
CARBOHYDRATES: 5G
PROTEIN: 5G

We hope that when you put this low-carb recipes booklet away, you've found a world of delicious treats that will tempt your taste senses and help you improve your health and well-being. We've welcomed the rich tastes, vivid colours, and healthful ingredients that make cooking low-carb an absolute pleasure throughout these dishes.

Every meal, from filling dinners to substantial breakfasts that start your day, was thoughtfully created to nourish your body and spirit. There are plenty of different alternatives to fit your tastes and dietary requirements, whether your goals are weight reduction, better metabolic health, or just a fresh appreciation for tasty, nutrient-dense food.

Beyond the kitchen, however, we want this cookbook to give you the information, motivation, and assurance you need to apply the low-carb lifestyle to your everyday life. You now possess the information and resources to succeed on your health path, from choosing what to eat to learning basic culinary skills.

As you delve further into low-carb cooking, remember that your enthusiasm for delicious food and health is the most vital component. Above all, enjoy feeding your family and yourself healthful, tasty meals. Pay attention to your body. Experiment with new tastes and ingredients.

We are grateful you could come along on this gastronomic journey. May these dishes fill your table with happiness, energy, and plenty both now and for many meals to come. To enjoy life's flavours, one delectable mouthful at a time.

happy cooking!